Bioceramics in Hip Joint Replacement

Bioceramics in Hip Joint Replacement

Proceedings 5th International CeramTec Symposium, Febr. 18/19, 2000

Edited by
Gerd Willmann, Karl Zweymüller

125 figures
25 tables

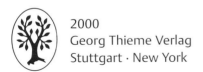

2000
Georg Thieme Verlag
Stuttgart · New York

Die Deutsche Bibliothek –
CIP-Einheitsaufnahme

Bioceramics in hip joint replacement :
proceedings ; Febr. 18/19, 2000
(G. Willmann ; K. Zweymüller. –
Stuttgart ; New York : Thieme, 2000
(... International CeramTec symposium... ; 5)

© 2000 Georg Thieme Verlag
Rüdigerstraße 14
70469 Stuttgart

Printed in Germany

Umschlaggestaltung:
S. Killinger, Kornwestheim
Satz: Ziegler + Müller, Kirchentellinsfurt
   Satzsystem: 3B2 (6.05)
Druck: Grammlich, Pliezhausen
Buchbinder: Held, Rottenburg

ISBN 3-13-105531-6   1 2 3 4 5 6

Wichtiger Hinweis: Wie jede Wissenschaft ist die Medizin ständigen Entwicklungen unterworfen. Forschung und klinische Erfahrung erweitern unsere Erkenntnisse, insbesondere was Behandlung und medikamentöse Therapie anbelangt. Soweit in diesem Buch eine Dosierung oder eine Applikation erwähnt wird, darf der Leser zwar darauf vertrauen, dass Autoren, Herausgeber und Verlag große Sorgfalt darauf verwandt haben, dass diese Angabe **dem Wissensstand bei Fertigstellung des Buches** entspricht.

Für Angaben über Dosierungsanweisungen und Applikationsformen kann vom Verlag jedoch keine Gewähr übernommen werden. **Jeder Benutzer ist angehalten,** durch sorgfältige Prüfung der Beipackzettel der verwendeten Präparate und gegebenenfalls nach Konsultation eines Spezialisten festzustellen, ob die dort gegebene Empfehlung für Dosierungen oder die Beachtung von Kontraindikationen gegenüber der Angabe in diesem Buch abweicht. Eine solche Prüfung ist besonders wichtig bei selten verwendeten Präparaten oder solchen, die neu auf den Markt gebracht worden sind. **Jede Dosierung oder Applikation erfolgt auf eigene Gefahr des Benutzers.** Autoren und Verlag appellieren an jeden Benutzer, ihm etwa auffallende Ungenauigkeiten dem Verlag mitzuteilen.

Geschützte Warennamen werden **nicht** besonders kenntlich gemacht. Aus dem Fehlen eines solchen Hinweises kann also nicht geschlossen werden, dass es sich um einen freien Warennamen handelt.

Das Buch, einschließlich aller seiner Teile ist urheberrechtlich geschützt. Jede Verwertung außerhalb der engen Grenzen des Urheberrechtsgesetzes ist ohne Zustimmung des Verlages unzulässig und strafbar. Das gilt insbesondere für Vervielfältigungen, Übersetzungen, Mikroverfilmungen und die Einspeicherung und Verarbeitung in elektronischen Systemen.

List of First Authors, President and Chairmen

President
Prim. Univ. – Prof. Dr. med. K. Zweymüller

Chairmen
Dr. M. Buttermilch
Dr. J. P. Garino
Dr. A. Toni
Prim. Univ.-Prof. Dr. med. K. Zweymüller

CeramTec Award 2000: Jury
Prof. Dr. med. H.-W. Springorum
   (Bad Mergentheim)
Prof. Dr. med. D. Stock (Braunschweig)
PD Dr. rer. nat. G. Willmann (CeramTec)
Prof. Dr. med. L. Zichner (Frankfurt/Main)

Authors
Dipl.-Ing. R. Bader (Arzt)
Hauptstraße 27/1
73102 Birenbach, Germany

Dr. Barahona
Policlinico Vigo S. A.
Salamanco, 5
36211 Vigo, Spain

J. Black, PhD, FBSE
Professional Consultation in
Biomaterials and Orthopaedic Engineering
409 Dorothy Drive
King of Prussia, PA 19406, USA

Prof. Franco Bonicoli
Primario Divisione Ortopedica
Ospedale di Lucca
Loc. Campo di Marte
55100 Lucca, Italy

J. M. Buchanan FRCS
13 Westfield Avenue
Gosforth
Newcastle Upon Tyne
Tyne & Wear, NE3 4 YH, U.K.

Dr. med. M. Buttermilch
CeramTec AG
Fabrikstr. 23 – 29
73207 Plochingen, Germany

Prof. Dr. med. C. Dietschi
Centro Orthopedica Nassa
Via Nassa 46
6900 Lugano, Switzerland

Prof. Dr. med. G. A. Fuchs
Klinikum Bayreuth
Preuschwitzer Str. 101
95445 Bayreuth, Germany

J. P. Garino MD
Assistant Professor
University of Pennsilvania,
School of Medicine
Department of Orthopedic Surgery
3400 Spruce Street, Silverstein Two
Philadelphia, PA 19104.4283, USA

PD Dr. med. Ch. Hendrich
Orthopädische Universitätsklinik
König-Ludwig-Haus
Brettreichstr. 11
97074 Würzburg, Germany

Dr. Ch. Kaddick
ENDO LAB
Isarstraße 1c
83026 Rosenheim, Germany

Dr. med. Ch. Lhotka
Schalkgasse 2/30
1180 Vienna, Austria

H. A. Mc Kellop, PhD
Biomechanical Lab. Dep. of Orthopaedics
Orthop. Hospital and University
of Southern California
2400 South Flower Street
Los Angeles, CA 9007, USA

Prof. Dr. Philippe Maury
Hôpital La Peyronie
371, av du doyen G. Giraud
34295 Montpellier Cedex 5, France

Prof. Dr. David G. Mendes
46 Kamil. Hoismans ST
Haifa, Israel

Dipl. Ing. H.-G. Pfaff
CeramTec AG
Fabrikstr. 23 – 29
73207 Plochingen, Germany

Dr. med. U. Pfeiffer
Orthopädische Klinik
Marienkrankenhaus
An St. Swidbert 17
40489 Düsseldorf-Kaiserswerth, Germany

PD Dr. med. R. P. Pitto
Orthopädische Universitätsklinik
und Poliklinik
Waldkrankenhaus St. Marien
Rathsbergerstraße 57
91054 Erlangen, Germany

Dipl. Ing. R. Rack
CeramTec AG
Fabrikstr. 23 – 29
73207 Plochingen, Germany

Dipl. Ing. J. Richter
Am Steg 1
89231 Neu-Ulm, Germany

PD Dr. med. G. Scheller
Oberarzt der Orthopädischen Klinik
Fakultät für klinische Medizin Mannheim
der Universität Heidelberg
Theodor Kutzer-Ufer 1 – 3
68167 Mannheim, Germany

Dr. med. E. Seeber
Chefarzt des Städt. Klinikums Dessau
Orthopädische Klinik
Schwabestr. 4
06846 Dessau, Germany

Dr. med. P. Thomas
Dermatologische Klinik und Poliklinik
Ludwig-Maximilians-Universität
Frauenlobstr. 9 – 11
80337 München, Germany

Dr. A. Toni
Laboratorio di Tecnologia dei Materiali
Istituti Orthopedici Rizzoli
via di Barbiano 1/10
40136 Bologna, Italy

Dr. J.-P. Vidalain
Clinique du lac et Argonnay
22, rue André Theuriet
74000 Annecy, France

PD Dr. rer. nat. G. Willmann
CeramTec AG
Fabrikstr. 23 – 29
73207 Plochingen, Germany

Prim. Univ.-Prof. Dr. med. K. Zweymüller
Ärztl. Direktor und Vorstand der
2. Orthopäd. Abteilung
KAV – Orthopäd. Krankenhaus Gersthof
Wielemansgasse 28
1180 Vienna, Austria

Foreword Proc 5th Int. CeramTec Symposium 2000

There is consensus that ceramics for bearing surfaces in total joint arthroplasty offer the option to reduce wear debris and to solve the problem of particle induced osteolysis.

I think that one of the most important achievements is the cooperation between engineers and surgeons. The development of bearing surfaces for joint replacements with ceramics started in the seventies. Ceramics proved to work, nevertheless there is still research ongoing all over the world. One of the objectives of the CeramTec Symposium is and always will be to compile results of clinical studies, technical research, and material developments. It is the objective to share all this with the orthopedic community. All the future Symposiums will be held in Stuttgart, Germany once a year.

Proceedings will be published right after the meetings. The Proceedings of the previous Symposiums are not available any more. Therefore CeramTec has copied all the previous Proceedings on a CD-ROM. The CD-ROM will be available in spring 2000. The Proceeding of the 5th Symposium will be available in summer 2000. I hope that the 5th Proceedings will provide a review and an update of ceramics in joint replacement for those who work in this field.

Prof. W. Puhl (Germany) was the President of the symposiums in 1996, 1997, and 1998. He had proposed that the future Presidents should be surgeons from other countries than Germany to underline that the Symposium is really an international one. Prof. L. Sedel (France) was the President of the 4th Symposium in 1999. I was honored when Prof. K. Zweymüller (Austria) had accepted to be the President of this Symposium. Dr. Aldo Toni (Italy) has agreed to be the President of the 6th Symposium scheduled for March 23/24 in 2001.

It has become a tradition that at the occasion of CeramTec's Symposium CeramTec awards a prize for outstanding studies with regard to the problems of wear in joint arthroplasty. This year's price was given to J. E. Nevelos (Leeds, U.K.) for a paper about investigations with a hip simulator. Members of the jury had been Prof. Springorum, Prof. Stock, and Prof. Zichner and me. The winner of the previous four awards had been from France, USA, and Germany. Again this proves that the CeramTec Symposium became an international event.

On this year's Symposium new topics have been discussed: Allergic reactions of biomaterials and the options of improved biomaterials, e.g. ceramic (bio-) composites.

I would like to thank Prof. Zweymüller, the speakers, the chairmen, the publisher Georg Thieme Verlag in Stuttgart, Germany, for the good discussions, their advice, help and support.

I would like to thank CeramTec's staff for all the good ideas and the support. My special thanks to the staff of the Interconti Hotel and Mr. A. Reindl for the excellent organization of this year's symposium.

March 2000   Gerd Willmann, MS PhD
Plochingen, Germany

Contents/Inhalt

1 Clinical Experience with Ceramics in Total Joint Replacement

1.1 Indikation und Kontraindikation für unterschiedliche Gleitpaarungen bei modularen Hüftpfannen 2
K. Zweymüller

1.2 Ten Rules of Technique for Ceramic Bearing Surfaces in Total Hip Arthroplasty 9
D. G. Mendes, M. Said, V. Zukerman

1.3 Early Experience with Alumina/Alumina Bearings in Hydroxyapatite Ceramic Total Hip Arthroplasty 12
J. M. Buchanan, A. Malcolm

1.4 Hip HA-Coated Prostheses and Ceramic-on-Ceramic Bearing Surface – A Reliable Solution for Young Patients ... 14
J.-P. Vidalain

1.5 Why Selecting the Ceramic on Ceramic Bearing Couple? 16
Ph. Maury, E. Gagneux, F. Gautier, S. Didelot

1.6 Modular Press-Fit Acetabular Components in Total Hip Arthroplasty ... 19
R. P. Pitto, D. Schwämmlein, M. Schramm

1.7 Klinische Erfahrungen und Migrationsanalyse – PLASMACUP 26
C. Hendrich, M. Blanke, U. Sauer, C. P. Rader, J. Eulert

1.8 MPF Modular Press Fit Cup – The Concept, Experience and First Results 35
G. Scheller, A. Claus, B. Günther, H. Schroeder-Boersch, L. Jani

1.9 2–4 Year Clinical Results with a Ceramic-on-Ceramic Articulation in a New Modular THR-System 39
G. A. Fuchs

1.10 Peri-Acetabular Osteolysis in Press-Fit Ceramic-Ceramic and Ceramic-Polyethylene Total Hip Replacement: 5–7 Years Follow-Up 46
F. Bonicoli

1.11 Do Ceramic Liners Alter the Load Transmission of Modular Hip Sockets? 54
C. Hendrich, C. Kaddick, H. G. Pfaff, G. Willmann

1.12 Acetabular Ceramic Insert Breakage in Total Hip Prostheses 64
D. Rueda, F. Barahona

2 Reliability – Clinical and Technical Aspect

2.1 Einschränkung der Range of Motion von Hüftendoprothesen durch Design, Position und Pfannenabrieb 66
R. Bader, G. Willmann

2.2 Pre-Operative Planning in THR is a Must 75
C. Dietschi, D. Buehler

2.3 Besteht ein Risiko, wenn keramische Kugelköpfe bei Revisionsoperationen auf in situ belassene Schäfte aufgesetzt werden? 76
G. Willmann, H. G. Richter, J. Richter, E. Steinhauser

2.4 Untersuchung von explantierten BIOLOX® Köpfen: Analyse der metallischen Abdrücke in der konischen Bohrung 81
G. Willmann, A. Brodbeck, H. G. Richter

2.5 The Status and Early Results of Modern Ceramic-Ceramic Total Hip Replacement in the United States 88
J. P. Garino

3 Ion Release/Hypersensitivity/Allergic Reactions: A Problem in THR?

3.1 Hypersensitivity in THR: A Case Study ... 94
E. Seeber

3.2 Clinical Relevance of Allergological Tests in Total Joint Replacement 101
M. Schramm, R. P. Pitto

3.3 Whole-Blood Cobalt and Chromium Levels in Patients Managed with Total Hip Replacements Involving Different Metal-on-Metal Combinations 107
C. Lhotka, J. Steffan, K. Zhuber, T. Szekeres, K. Zweymüller

3.4 Biological Effects of Implanted Metallic Devices 112
J. Black, J. J. Jacobs

3.5 Allergological Aspects of Implant Biocompatibility 117
Peter Thomas, Munich, Germany

4 Advanced Materials for Bearing Surfaces in Joint Replacement

4.1 Simulator Testing of the Wear Couple ZTA-on-Polyethylene 124
A. Toni, S. Affatato, B. Bordini

4.2 New Generation Ceramics 127
G. Willmann

4.3 A New Material Concept for Bioceramics in Orthopedics 136
H.-G. Pfaff, R. Rack

4.4 A New Ceramic Material for Orthopaedics 141
R. Rack, H.-G. Pfaff

4.5 Wear Study in the Alumina-Zirconia System 146
C. Kaddick, H.-G. Pfaff

5 CeramTec Award 2000

5.1 CeramTec Award 2000 152

5.2 Wear of HIPed and Non-HIPed Alumina-Alumina Hip Joints Under Standard and Severe Simulator Testing Conditions 153
J. E. Nevelos, E. Ingham, C. Doyle, A. B. Nevelos, J. Fisher

5.3 CeramTec Award 1996–1999 154

6 Suggested Reading

6.1 Suggested Reading 156
G. Willmann

7 Workshop on the 5th Symposium

7.1 Workshop on the 5th Symposium 160
G. Willmann

1 Clinical Experience with Ceramics in Total Joint Replacement

1.1 Indikation und Kontraindikation für unterschiedliche Gleitpaarungen bei modularen Hüftpfannen

K. Zweymüller

Unsere Erfahrungen mit Keramikimplantaten zur Therapie der Coxarthrose reichen auf die Mitte der siebziger Jahre zurück. Damals verwendeten wir die sogenannte Metall-Keramik-Verbundendoprothese zur teilweise knochenzementfreien Implantation (13). Bei der Pfanne handelte es sich um eine keramische, monolithische Pfanne, deren Konstruktionsmerkmal drei Füßchen waren. Sie wurde ohne Knochenzement verankert. Eine keramische Kugel artikulierte mit dieser Pfanne. Die Verlaufsbeobachtungen zeigten eine fehlende Osteointegration dieser Pfanne mit sekundärer Cranialmigration, sowie auch Abriebprobleme zwischen den artikulierenden Oberflächen.

Im Jahre 1977 publizierten Semlitsch u. M. (11) Ergebnisse mit der Keramik-Polyäthylen-Artikulation von Hüftendoprothesen. Dabei zeigte sich, dass diese Kombination den herkömmlichen Metall-Polyäthylen-Artikulationen, was den Abrieb des Polyäthylens betraf, deutlich überlegen war. Simulatoruntersuchungen von Dowson u. M. zeigten Ähnliches im Vergleich zur Metall-Metall-Artikulation der Charnley Endoprothese (3). In-vivo-Untersuchungen der späteren Jahre, wie etwa von Zichner und Lindenfeld ergaben, dass nach einem Einlaufverschleiß, der etwa sechs Monate dauerte, und bis zu 0,5 mm per Jahr betrug, dieser Verschleiß nach einigen Jahren auf 0,1 mm bei Keramik-Polyäthylen-Artikulation und 0,2 mm bei Metall-Polyäthylen-Artikulation reduziert war (12).

Die Möglichkeit, den Polyäthylenabrieb zu verringern, war ausschlaggebend, eine Keramikkugel als Artikulationspartner unseres zementfreien Schaftes (erstmals implantiert Oktober 1979) zur Polyäthylen-Pfanne zu verwenden. Diese Pfanne, eine zementfreie Polyäthylen-Schraubpfanne (4,5), war ebenfalls eine monolithische Pfanne. Sie wurde im Hinblick auf eine gewisse Isoelastizität zum umgebenden knöchernen Pfannenlager, entsprechend den Basisarbeiten von C. Dietschi (2), eingeführt. Bekannterweise funktioniert jedoch eine Direktverankerung eines Polyäthylen-Implantates im Knochen nicht, da es zu massivem Abrieb des Polyäthylen kommt. Die Folge sind sekundäre Destruktionsprozesse des umgebenden Lagerknochens (9,10), egal, wie immer die Form und Oberfläche dieses Polyäthylens aussieht. Dies gilt auch für die metal-backed Pfannensysteme, bei denen Teile des Polyäthylen ungeschützt bleiben und somit in direkten Kontakt zum Knochen treten können.

Die erste modulare Pfannenkonstruktion eigener Entwicklung wurde Anfang 1985 eingeführt (15). Es handelte sich dabei um eine selbstschneidende Titan-Schraubpfanne mit einem Polyäthylen-Inlay. Gleitpartner dazu war eine Keramikkugel. Die Ergebnisse damit waren gut (1,6). Probleme gab es durch fallweise Überbeanspruchung des Polyäthylens vor allem dann, wenn eine 32 mm Keramikkugel in Kombination mit einer sehr kleinen Pfanne, d. h. mit sehr dünnem Polyäthylen-Inlay verwendet wurde. Es standen damals drei Halslängen für die Keramikkugel zur Verfügung, nämlich kurz, mittel und lang. Somit verfügten wir damals bereits über ein modulares System mit einer Vielzahl von Kombinationsmöglichkeiten.

Die Hauptanforderung an ein modernes Hüftendoprothesensystem ist die Verfügbarkeit unterschiedlichster Schaft- und Pfannengrößen sowie unterschiedlicher Halslängen. Ein Schaftsystem zur Durchführung von Primärimplantationen sollte um ein Revisionssystem erweitert werden, so dass ein modernes Prothesensystem nach dem Baukastenprinzip aufgebaut sein sollte. Damit kann die überwiegende Mehrzahl der Hüftgelenke, seien es Primär- seien es Revisionseingriffe versorgt werden. Für den Pfannenbereich gilt heute die absolute Forderung nach Modularität. Eine modulare Pfannenkonstruktion kann sich einer Sandwich-Technik mittels zwischengeschalteten Polyäthylen-Körpers zwischen einem Metall- oder Keramikinlay in der metallischen Pfannenschale bedienen, kann aber auch ein Keramikinlay in direkter Verankerung zur Metallschale anbieten.

Unsere Erfahrung mit konischen Schraubpfannen aus Reintitan erstreckt sich über 15 Jahre. Vor 7 Jahren wurde die durchgehend konische Pfannenform verlassen. Seither verwenden wir eine doppelkonische (bikonische) Schraubpfanne (14). Diese verfügt über die bekannten Vorteile einer konischen Pfanne, wie die Möglichkeit des Einbringens unter Vorspannung bei gleichzeitig minimaler Knochenresektion. Für die Hart-Hart-Artikulation eines Keramik-Inlay mit der Keramikkugel bedienen wir uns der Sandwich-Technik mit zwischengeschaltetem Polyäthylen. Die Frage, die heute immer wieder diskutiert wird ist die, ob ein zwischengeschaltetes Polyäthylen die Sicherheit des Implantates gefährden könnte. Dabei ist zu bedenken, dass die Exposition des Polyäthylen zur Umgebung in einem Sandwich-Design wesentlich geringer ist, als es in einer Keramik-Polyäthylen-Kombination gegeben ist. Zum anderen ist das Polyäthylen in einem Sandwich-Design keiner tribologischen Beanspruchung ausgesetzt, vorausgesetzt das Inlay ist stabil in der Pfannenschale verankert.

Während in der durchgehend konischen Schraubpfanne der ersten Generation, verwendet ab 1985, die Verankerung des Polyäthylen in der Pfannenschale noch nicht absolut stabil war, wurde der Verankerungsmechanismus in der bikonischen Pfanne deutlich verbessert. Durch einen Mehrfachkonus im Inneren der Pfannenschale wird das Polyäthylen so verankert, dass nun auch keinerlei Mikrobewegungen mehr möglich sind (14). Auf diese Weise scheint für uns das Problem des Polyäthylen-Abriebes in der Pfannenschale minimiert. Allerdings wissen wir nicht, ob es durch Alterungsvorgänge des Polyäthylens und somit durch Veränderungen der physikalischen Eigenschaften in etwa 15 bis 20 Jahren nicht doch zu Veränderungen kommt, die heute nicht voraussehbar sind.

Die intraoperativen Anforderungen an modulare Pfannen sind einerseits eine leichte Insertion aller Teile, andererseits aber auch eine leichte Entfernbarkeit der individuellen Teile im Falle von Revisionen (Abb. 7, 8). Auf Grund der Erkenntnisse von Huber und Lintner (8) hinsichtlich der Ausbreitung von Bakterienrasen auf keramischen Oberflächen ist im Falle von Revisionen bei Frühinfekten nicht nur das Inlay der Pfanne zu wechseln, sondern auch die Kugel. Die Metallschale sowie der Schaft können bei Frühinfekten durchaus belassen werden. Die Pfanne wäre infolge der raschen ossären Einbauvorgänge auch nur schwer herauszudrehen und kann nötigenfalls durch ein Zerschneiden in Segmente mittels eines Diamantfräsers entfernt werden.

Ein weiterer Vorteil eines Sandwich-Design ist die hohe Bruchfestigkeit eines Keramikinlays. In der von uns verwendeten Form beträgt diese weit mehr als 10 Tonnen, bei einer Minimalanforderung von 4,6 Tonnen. Diese wird nicht nur beim Sandwich-Design um ein Vielfaches überschritten, denn auch eine Konusfixation eines Keramikinlays ohne zwischengeschaltetes Polyäthylen hält mehr als 6 Tonnen beim Bersttest aus (Abb. 1).

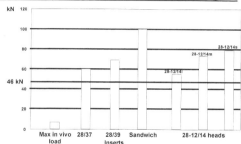

Abb. 1 Berstfestigkeit unterschiedlicher Materialkombinationen. Sie ist für die Sandwich-Konstruktion mit zwischengeschaltetem Polyäthylen mit 100 kN (10 Tonnen) am höchsten.

Während wir bei der Metall-Metall-Artikulation fünf verschiedene Halslängen, von S bis XXL zur Verfügung haben, waren es bei der Keramik bis vor drei Jahren nur drei. Seither verfügen wir noch über eine vierte Halslänge, nämlich die XL-Keramikkugel, deren besonderes Konstruktionsmerkmal ein pilzförmiger Kragen darstellt. Es ist jedoch zu bedenken, dass jede Art von Kragen, sei es bei Metallkugeln, sei es bei Keramikkugeln, eine deutliche Einschränkung des Bewegungsausmaßes darstellt (Abb. 4, 5). So beträgt das Bewegungsausmaß bei der von uns verwendeten Metall-Metall-Artikulation Standard bei Kugelkopfgröße L 126°, während es bei XXL nur 98° ausmacht (Abb. 2). Bei Verwendung von XL oder XXL Metallkugeln besteht deshalb, vor allem dann, wenn sie jüngeren Patienten eingebaut

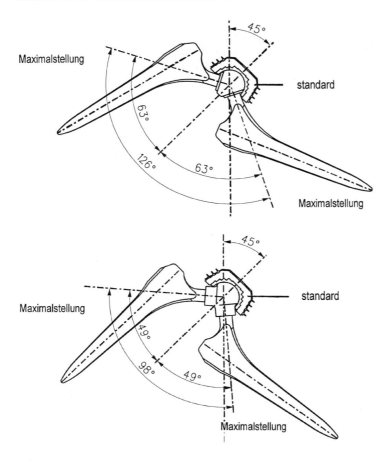

Abb. 2 a Die Bewegungsfreiheit der Metall-Metall-Artikulation mit Standard Inlay, Kugel L, Schaftgröße 5, Pfanne Größe 3.

b Die Bewegungsfreiheit der Metall-Metall-Artikulation mit Standard Inlay, Kugel XXL, Schaftgröße 5, Pfanne Größe 3.

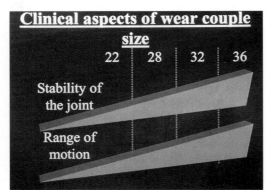

Abb. 3 Sowohl die Stabilität des Gelenkes gegen Luxation, als auch das Bewegungsausmaß sind bei Verwendung von Kugelkopfgröße 32 größer als bei einem Kugelkopf mit 28 mm Durchmesser.

werden, die Gefahr, dass es durch Kontakt des Kugelhalses mit dem Metallinlay zu Abrieb des Metalles und in weiterer Folge zu Metallose kommt (Abb. **7**). Die Gefahr des Kontaktes des Kugelhalses mit der Pfanne besteht auch bei Verwendung der XL Keramikkugel, bei der das Bewegungsausmaß noch weiter eingeschränkt ist (Abb. **5**). Wir sind deshalb der Ansicht, dass bei Primärimplantationen nach Möglichkeit keine XL oder XXL Kugelköpfe verwendet werden sollten. Allerdings, bei korrekter Implantation sämtlicher Teile und bei keinem übermäßigen Bewegungsausmaß sollte auch diese Möglichkeit durchaus in Betracht gezogen werden können. Niemals allerdings darf eine XL Keramikkugel dann verwendet werden, wenn sie gegen ein Keramikinlay läuft. Durch den Kontakt des Kugelkopfkragens mit dem Keramikinlay kann es zu Brüchen des Keramikinlays und somit zum Versagen des Systems kommen (Abb. **8**).

1.1 Indikation und Kontraindikation für unterschiedliche Gleitpaarungen

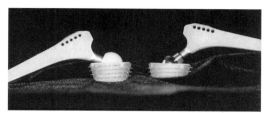

Abb. 4 Das Bewegungsausmaß einer Metallkugel mit XXL-Halslänge ist signifikant geringer gegenüber einer Standard-Keramikkugel.

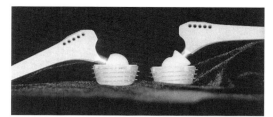

Abb. 5 Das Bewegungsausmaß einer Keramikkugel mit XL-Halslänge ist signifikant geringer gegenüber einer Standard-Keramikkugel sowie auch gegenüber einer XXL-Metallkugel (s. a. Abb. **4**).

Tab. 1 Impingement in XL and XXL ball heads

Ceramic-Ceramic	Breakage
Ceramic-Polyethylene	PE wear → Osteolysis
Metal-Metal	Metal wear → Osteolysis
Metal-Polyethylene	PE wear → Osteolysis

Eine eingeschränkte Bewegungsfunktion seitens der Implantate birgt somit immer die Gefahr eines Impingments in sich. XL und XXL Kugelköpfe können ein Impingement verursachen, deren Folge die Stabilität der Implantate gefährden (Tab. **1**).

Neben der Konstruktion des Kugelkopfes gibt es jedoch noch andere Ursachen für ein Impingement, nämlich exzessive Bewegungsausschläge, die Konstruktion des Kugelkopfes, die Konstruktion der Pfanne, eine Fehlposition der Komponenten sowie auch anatomische Gegebenheiten. Letztere können belassene Osteophyten im Bereiche des Acetabulums sein, sowie auch die Konfiguration des proximalen ventralen Femur. Ist dieses nämlich besonders prominent ausgeprägt, so kann es bei belassenen Pfannenosteophyten bei

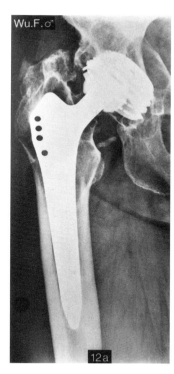

Abb. 6
a Männlich, 63 Jahre. 12 Jahre nach Implantation einer Titanium-Pfannenschale sowie eines Titaniumgeradschafts („Alloclassic"). Deutliches Aufbrauchen des Polyäthylen-Inlays cranial. Ausgeprägte paraartikuläre Ossifikationen, welche eine strenge Limitierung der Außenrotation bewirkten.

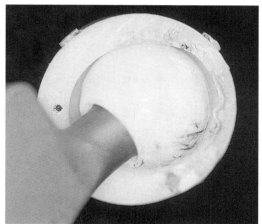

b Durch das Anpressen des Keramikkugelkopfes an das Polyäthylen-Inlay bei jeder Außenrotation ist es durch dieses extraartikulär bedingte Impingement zu einem frühzeitigen Abrieb des Inlays gekommen.

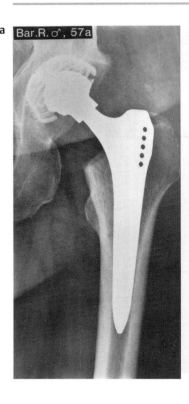
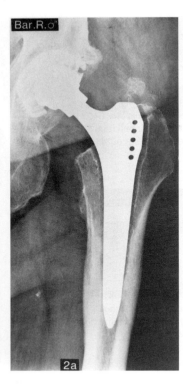

Abb. 7 a Männlich, 57 Jahre. Ersatz des linken Hüftgelenkes durch eine zementfreie Titaniumpfanne sowie durch einen Titanium-Geradschaft (Plus-Endoprothetik). Metall-Metall-Artikulation mit Verwendung eines XXL- Kugelkopfes. Reguläre Position der Implantate postoperativ.
b 2 Jahre postoperativ. Infolge einer ausgeprägten Osteolyse um das Implantat Lockerung des Titaniumschaftes.
c Monitorgezielte ap-Aufnahme der Pfanne. Metall-Metall-Artikulation mit Antiluxationsinlay. Die Titanium-Pfannenschale ist stabil im Knochen verankert.

Flexion und vor allem Innenrotation des Beines zu einem Impingement, gefolgt von einer Luxation der Kugel nach dorsal zu kommen. Ein besonderer Fall eines Impingement kann durch Bewegungseinschränkung durch paraartikuläre Ossifikationen gegeben sein. Durch einen harten Anschlag bei der Außenrotation kann es zu Überlastungen des Polyäthylen-Inlays kommen (Abb. **6**).

Bei Revisionsfällen, vor allem bei älteren Patienten stehen wir der Verwendung einer XL Keramikkugel oder XL- oder XXL-Metallkugel aber durchaus positiv gegenüber. Dies vor allem deshalb, weil es ja bei diesen Patienten doch zu einer Limitation der Beweglichkeit und vor allem auch der Aktivität gekommen ist. Trotzdem ist infolge des geringeren Bewegungsausmaßes immer an eine tendenziell erhöhte Luxationsbereitschaft zu denken.

Ein Impingment verursacht eine hohe Druckbelastung auf einem relativ kleinen Areal, somit eine punktförmige Belastung. Diese punktförmige Belastung kann, vor allem dann, wenn diese im Rahmen einer Subluxation bei Keramik-Keramik-Kombination auftritt, zu Abrieb führen. Im Falle

d
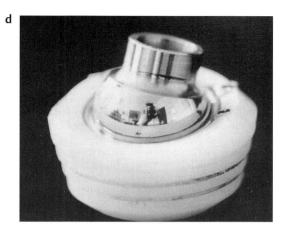

e
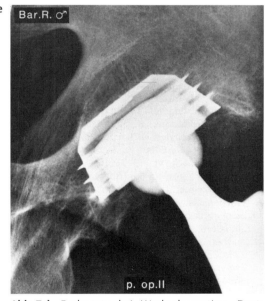

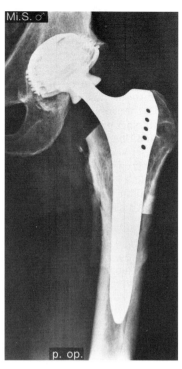

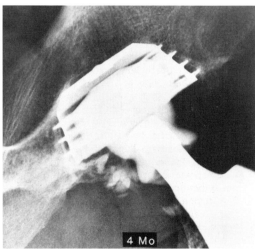

Abb. 8 a Männlich, 45 Jahre. Ersatz des linken Hüftgelenkes durch eine zementfreie Titaniumpfanne sowie durch einen Titanium-Geradschaft (Plus-Endoprothetik). Keramik-Keramik-Artikulation mit Verwendung eines XL-Keramik-Kugelkopfes. Reguläre Position der Implantate postoperativ.

Abb. 7 d Explantate bei Wechseloperation. Deutliche Schlifffurche am Kragen des XXL-Kugelkopfes, verursacht durch ein Impingement mit dem Metall-Pfanneninlay. Als Folge des Metallabschliffes deutliche Metallose, gefolgt von der Lockerung des Schaftimplantates. **e** Monitorgezielte ap-Aufnahme. Zustand nach Revisionseingriff. Das Polyäthylen-Metallinlay wurde gegen ein Polyäthylen-Keramikinlay gewechselt. Die Titanium-Pfannenschale wurde belassen.

mehrfacher postoperativer Luxationen bei Verwendung einer Keramik-Keramik-Paarung empfehlen wir die Reoperation des Patienten. Dabei sollte das Keramikinlay entfernt werden und entweder durch ein neues Inlay, besser aber durch ein

b Monitorgezielte ap-Aufnahme, 4 Monate postoperativ. Ausgeprägte röntgendichte Verschattungen um den caudalen Kopf- und Pfannenanteil: durch das Impingement der Kragenpartie des Kopfes ist es zu einem Ausbruch des keramischen Pfanneninlays gekommen. Das Inlay sowie der Kopf wurden daraufhin gewechselt und durch eine Keramik-Polyäthylen-Kombination ersetzt. Die Pfannenschale war stabil und wurde belassen.

Polyäthylen-Inlay ersetzt werden. Zur Reduktion der Luxationsbereitschaft kann weiters anstelle einer 28er Kugel eine Kugel mit 32 mm Durchmesser Anwendung finden. Ein Kugelkopf Größe 32 verringert auch dadurch, dass mit ihm größere Bewegungsausmaße möglich sind, die Gefahr eines Impingment und somit die einer postoperativen Luxation (Abb. **3**). Da gerade bei älteren Patienten die Häufigkeit einer postoperativen Luxation (7) erhöht ist, sind Überlegungen, bei dieser Patientengruppe von der Verwendung der 28 mm Kugel auf 32 mm überzugehen, durchaus angezeigt. Sowohl das größere Bewegungsausmaß als auch die höhere Stabilität der Kugel gegenüber Luxationen sprechen in diese Richtung.

Literatur

1 Delaunay C. P., Kapandji A. I. (1996) Primary Total Hip Arthroplasty with the Karl Zweymüller First-Generation Cementless Prosthesis (A 5- to 9-Year Retrospective Study). J Arthroplasty, Vol. 11, No. 6: 643–652.
2 Dietschi C. (1978) Experimentelle Untersuchungen zum Kraftfluß an Becken und Hüftazetabulum und deren Bedeutung für den künstlichen Hüftgelenkpfannenersatz. In: Zur Problematik des künstlichen Hüftgelenks. Eichler J. (Hrsg.): Schriftenreihe der Medizinisch-Orthopädischen Technik, Bd. 3.
3 Dowson D., Jobbins B., Seyed-Harraf A. (1993) An evaluation of the penetration of ceramic femoral heads into polyethylene acetabular cups. Wear, 162–164: 880–889.
4 Endler M., Endler F. (1982) Theoretisch-experimentelle Grundlagen und erste klinische Erfahrungen mit einer neuen zementfreien Polyäthylenschraubpfanne bei Hüftgelenksersatz. Acta Chirurgica Austriaca, Suppl. 45.
5 Endler M., Endler F., Plenk H. (1983) Experimentelle Aspekte und klinische Früherfahrungen einer zementlosen Hüftgelenkpfanne aus UHMW-Polyäthylen. In: Morscher E. (Hrsg.): Die zementlose Fixation von Hüftendoprothesen. Springer, Berlin, Heidelberg, New York, Tokyo.
6 Eyb R., Kutschera H. P., Schartelmueller T., Toma C., Zweymüller K. (1993) Mid Term Experience With the Cementless Zweymüller System. Results of a Minimum Five-Year-Follow-up Study. Acta Orthop Belg, 59, Suppl 1: 138–143.
7 Grossmann P., Braun M., Becker W. (1994) Luxationen nach Hüft-TEP-Implantationen. Z. Orthop. 132: 521–526.
8 Huber M., Lintner F. (1999) Bacterial adhesion to femoral ball head surfaces of artificial hip joints in vitro. Eur J Orthop Surg Traumatol. 9: 245–250.
9 Lintner F., Böhm G., Bösch P., Brand G., Endler M., Zweymüller K. (1990) Results of histological and microradiographic examination of cementless implanted polyethylene threaded hip sockets. In. Willert H. G., Buchhorn G. H., Eyerer D. (Hrsg.): Ultra-High Molecular Weight Polyethylene as Biomaterial in Orthopedic Surgery. Hogrefe-Huber, Toronto, New York, Bern, Göttingen, Stuttgart.
10 Lintner F., Böhm G., Brand G., Endler M., Zweymüller K. (1988) Ist hochdichtes Polyäthylen als Implantatmaterial zur zementfreien Verankerung von Hüftendoprothesen geeignet? Eine histomorphologische Untersuchung an explantierten Polyäthylenschraubpfannen. Z. Orthop. 126: 688–692.
11 Semlitsch M., Lehmann M., Weber H., Doerre E., Willert H. G. (1977) New prospects for a prolonged functional life-span of artificial hip joints by using the material combination polyethylene/aluminium oxide ceramic/metal. J Biomed Mater Res, 11: 537–552.
12 Zichner L., Lindenfeld T. (1997) In-vivo-Verschleiß der Gleitpaarungen Keramik-Polyethylen gegen Metall-Polyethylen. Orthopäde, 26: 129–134.
13 Zweymüller K., Chiari K., Salzer M., Plenk H. jr, Punzet G., Locke H. (1977) Eine Metall-Keramik-Verbundprothese für das Hüftgelenk zur teilweise knochenzementfreien Implantation. Wien. Klin. Wochenschr., 89: 462
14 Zweymüller K., Deckner A., Kupferschmidt W., Steindl M. (1994) Die Weiterentwicklung der konischen Schraubpfanne. Med. Ortho. Tech. 114: 223–228.
15 Zweymüller K., Lintner F., Semlitsch M. (1988) Biologic Fixation of a Press-Fit Titanium Hip Joint Endoprosthesis. Clin Orthop. 235: 195–206.

1.2 Ten Rules of Technique for Ceramic Bearing Surfaces in Total Hip Arthroplasty

D. G. Mendes, M. Said, V. Zukerman

The tribological properties favors ceramic articulating surfaces as the preferred technology for future orthopaedic implants. But, there are points of concern that we have to recognize and face. If we adequately care for them, this will give us confidence in performing the surgical procedures for the full benefit of the patients and for the longest durability of the implants.

I shall mention three points of concern. Wear remains our long term main concern. The volume of wear and the size and shape of the particles affects the tissue reaction which depends on the extent of the body rejection phenomenon as well. This is the main cause for loosening of the implant. To reduce wear to a minimum, the choice of ceramics seems to be justified by present clinical experience. Indeed a few of the rules that I shall discuss relate to reduction of wear. Stress shielding of the host bone because of stiffness, also is a long term concern, but is not in the scope of this paper.

Indeed our immediate main concern is fragility. In the United States ceramics are considered fragile. Are they fragile also in Europe and Israel? To answer this question negatively, a meticulous, unforgiving and reproducible surgical technique is required. Therefore we have formulated essential rules of proper technique and included: accurate fit of the components, accurate orientation of the components, stability of the joint, adequate tissue tension, caring for debris and prevention of metal transfer due to ceramic–metal touch. I would like to acknowledge the paper by Dr J. Gekeler on the same subject in 1998 (1).

Ten is our traditional number for setting up rules. I shall use this number for setting the rules of "do" and "do not". These ten rules strictly guide the surgeon toward achieving durability and longevity of the implant.

Rules of "DO"

1 Osseo-Integration

The indication for use of ceramic articulation for young patients rely on the superior tribological properties of ceramics. In young age, fixation of hip joint prosthetic components is generally done without cement by osseo-integration. We have had excellent long term experience in using Mathys coated acetabular cups. Coating was either with hydroxyapatite granules or titanium powder.

Eventually we have used Morscher cups with Sulzer titanium mesh.

Likewise we have had excellent long term experience with Landos femoral stems of titanium alloy coated with hydroxy-apatite. Presently we use a combination of Aesculap Plasma cups and Landos hydroxy-apatite stems as the components that bear the Biolox-Forte alumina articulation surfaces.

2 Press fit

Osseo-integration is achieved by press fit of the implant components within the center of the available bone. Reaming is carried deep into the acetabulum to have it deeper than wider. Thus the cup is pressed around its periphery by the border of the acetabulum, mainly between the anterior and posterior bony rims. Screws are avoided and not used except for special cases such as in revisions. The strength of the fit is assessed at surgery by maneuvering the introducer and by strong push with an impactor on the medial rim of the metal back plasma cup.

The stem of our choice is fixed by press fit in its proximal part. This is ascertained at surgery by applying torque on the stem. Being a tapered stem design, the acting compressive forces tend to increase its purchase in bone and promote stability. Bending and torque moments are resisted by the circumferential fit of the stem in bone.

3 Perfect Adaptation of Components

Ceramics are highly sensitive to stress raisers which may crack the material. Therefore, the technology of surface finish and perfect conformity and fit is of the highest quality. Two systems of Morse taper cone make the structural design for the bearing components of the implant: the alumina head over the neck taper cone and the alumina insert inside the cup taper cone. The required perfect fit does not allow any particles of debris in the opposing areas of contact, neither bony debris nor soft tissue.

4 Components Orientation

The stability of coupled ceramic components is essential, more so than with coupling of other materials. Polyethylene and metals are more forgiving to impacts, such as in complications of recurrent subluxation or in dislocation and reduction. With ceramics the risk of chipping and breakage is high, therefore stability cannot be compromised. For a stable joint appropriate orientation of the components must be achieved. These are strictly set by the theta angle of the cup and by the alpha anteversion angles of the cup and the stem. X ray control during surgery may be used to ascertain these positions.

Stability of the joint is ascertained at the end of surgery by having unrestricted full range of motion. With a stable joint done through anterolateral approach the patient is allowed to perform the full range of Praying Exercises for regaining motion the day after surgery.

5 Soft Tissue Tension

Adequate soft tissue tension holds the joint together and keeps it stable. Soft tissue tension is controlled by careful planning of the levels of bony cuts, and proper relaxation given by the anaesthetist during reduction. In special cases such as high dislocated hips or revision surgery, when muscle imbalance is accompanied with contractures, osteotomy and reattachment of either the greater or lesser trochanter or both is required to restores appropriate muscle balance.

Rules of "DO NOT"

6 Narrow Angle Load

The need for reduction of rate of wear and the relative fragility at the periphery of ceramic components require that loads should be transferred by large areas of contact. Narrow angle load decreases contact areas and increases contact stresses, therefore must be avoided. Narrow angle load results from badly oriented components (Fig. 1). Mainly due to high theta angle, insufficient alpha angle of anteversion or excessive anteversion. It is particularly during activities in flexion, such as raising from a chair or climbing stairs, that load is high and mal orientation in a narrow angles exposes the head to higher stresses.

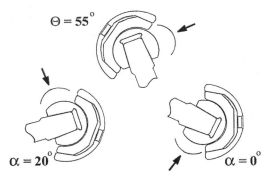

Fig. 1 Diagrammatic presentation of narrow angle loads due to mal position of components.

7 Edge Loading

Edge loading is more characteristic in Knee Arthroplasty. In the hip it may result from temporary positions in the case of subluxation or dislocation (Fig. 2). It is a harmful situation and may cause chipping and breakage of the ceramic.

8 Impingement

Impingement upon the components is critical. This occurs mainly due to mal-orientation (Fig. 3). It may result as well from having a narrow offset of the femur, due to a small head and neck or high neck shaft angle. Low theta angle causes impingement in abduction. Retroversion or neutral anteversion cause impingement in

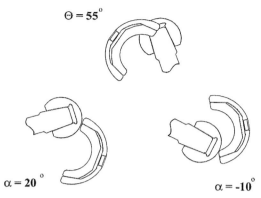

Fig. 2 Diagrammatic presentation of edge loading due to subluxation and dislocation.

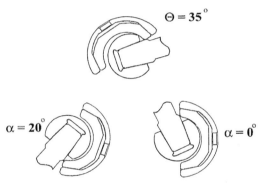

Fig. 3 Diagrammatic presentation of Impingement due to mal-position of components.

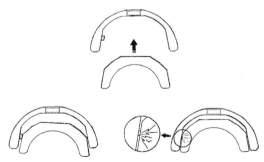

Fig. 4 Diagrammatic presentation of particle entrapment causing a point of stress raiser.

flexion. Excessive anteversion causes impingement in extension and external rotation.

The periphery of the ceramic insert of the cup is particularly in danger because of impingement with the metal neck, but the ceramic head may also be in jeopardy. Impingement may cause chipping and nock off large fragments of ceramics.

9 Stress Raisers

Stress raisers are important to be recognized and avoided. They may result from imperfect production of the taper cones systems, from re-use of used cones as in case of revision surgery and from mishandling of the system. During surgery, awareness of particles which may cause three body wear are an important rule to prevent entrapped stress raisers (Fig. 4).

10 Metal Powder Transfer

Transfer of metal powder to the ceramic surface is not adequately recognized. It may happen not UN-frequently during surgery at any time that metallic instrument or implant touches the ceramic surface. It may also happen by the use of retractors or impactors and during trial and final reduction. Metallic transfer is easily recognized by blackish areas or spots which feel rough to finger touch. It spoils the smoothness of the ceramic surface finish and can be removed only by treatment with highly strong acid.

I have presented ten rules and assume that with your vast experience you may have set for yourself further rules, that I am willing to learn.

Finally, I have left a few open questions for further discussion:
1. What is the diameter of choice for ceramic bearings? Is it different from articulation with polyethylene?
2. Is it justified in certain cases with poor bone stock to ream through the medial wall in-order to achieve stable press fit?
3. Would it be a proper recommendation to have routine fluoroscopy control for positioning of the cup?
4. Are we satisfied of the available modalities to accurately measure wear of the articulation surfaces and displacement of the components?

Reference

1 Gekeler J. In: The Bicontact Hip Implant System, Georg Thieme Verlag, Stuttgart, New York, 1998

1.3 Early Experience with Alumina/Alumina Bearings in Hydroxyapatite Ceramic Total Hip Arthroplasty

J. M. Buchanan, A. Malcolm

Thank you for inviting me come to talk to you about my experience with ceramic on ceramic bearing surfaces in hip surgery. I have been using HA coated hip implants for over eleven years with satisfactory results. As a sub group I have a series of hips with ceramic bearings.

I have always been concerned about the deterioration of cemented hips after about 8, 9 or ten years. They get progressively more stiff and x-rays show loosening at the cement/bone interface. More worryingly they present with granulomatous deposits around the implants with obvious bone destruction. Histology shows macrophages laden with cement and polyethylene debris. Gruen and others have reported that polythene wear causes the release of between half a million and a million particles each step.

The current problems of hip arthroplasty are thus generated by using cement and polythene.

Avoiding these materials should lengthen the useful life of the replaced hip.

I have been using Hydroxyapatite Ceramic coated implants since 1988. There is no cement and the implants are anchored by bone integrating with the HA layer. I have used alumina ceramic heads since the beginning and ceramic on ceramic bearings in younger patients since October 1991. Some implants are available after death. Histology of undecalcified sections of HA coated implants shows that cancellous bone bonds to the HA coating within six weeks. It is also evident that HA will be replaced with bone by the natural process of osteoclastic and osteoblastic bone substitution over a period of several years. However the HA is replaced with bone but without any intervening fibrous tissue. This should be better than cement and obviates the risk of granulomatous disease from the cement.

Ceramic on ceramic bearings provide a smooth surface with little expected development of wear debris. This relies on accurate manufacture of the implants with truly round heads and round acetabula. I am not an expert on ceramics but I understand that spherical deviation is of the order of 1000 Angstroms which equates to 150 unit cells of the alumina crystal lattice.

Surface finish is paramount and the Hot Isostatic Postcompaction or HIP process helps achieve astonishing smoothness. Alumina heads treated this way and examined with dye under $100 \times$ magnification show no pores. A laser microscope shows a surface profile with a homogenous distribution of very small deviations.

My principal experience is with alumina although I have inserted some Zirconia heads.

The alumina is relatively brittle and needs to be supported in the acetabulum. An early design had a raised edge which was unsupported and has broken off in one of my hips. The newer design has removed this lip and I have seen no more fractures. There may be a limit on patient weight and I have seen one ceramic liner fracture in a man of 23 stone (146 Kilos).

At an anecdotal level these hips work well and with the short follow up that I have, they all perform as well as any other hip. I feel that young patients, that is those who have a life expectancy of 20 years or more, should be offered ceramic on ceramic hips to obviate polythene debris and the granulomata it produces.

This young lady who is only 42 now had her hip replaced 8 years ago. She is catching up on lost time playing with her children and really does more than I would like on her hip. Road running was on the list but she now limits herself to mountain walking and trampolining.

This man who is now 56 had both his hips replaced nearly six years ago. Not only is he a black belt at Karate but he teaches it at night school.

Results

Out of a total of 1380 hips in my Hydroxyapatite series, 179 of them have ceramic/ceramic bearings. These are in 163 patients, 16 have had bilateral operations. There are more men than women in this relatively young group of patients.

You will see the age range with the youngest at 19 and the eldest at 66 with a mean age of 47.

Follow-up

The table shows the length of follow up. You will note 4 hips over 8 years and a total of 45 hips followed for more than 5 years. None have been lost to follow up. There has been one death from heart disease at 4 years.

Indications

You will see from the list that 84 had osteoarthritis, 12 had rheumatoid arthritis and 12 had ankylosing spondylitis. 11 had avascular necrosis. 30 of them had hip dysplasia and 7 had had CDH.

Assessment

All the patients are assessed with the Harris Hip Score (HSS) pre-operatively and post-operatively. They are seen at 3 months, 6 months and 12 months. They are then reviewed annually.

Preoperative HHS shows that they are all disabled many scoring in the 10, 20, 30 range.

Post operatively 128 out of 171 score between 90 and 100.

Of 171 hips followed up more than 3 months, the Harris Hip Score was less than 80 in 20 patients.

Of these 20 patients with a low Harris Hip Score, 12 were pain free but had other joint or medical problems. This left 8 patients with poor Harris Hip Scores and poor pain scores.

The problem patients included 2 with infection, two fractured ceramic liners and four other patients.

Complications

Two patients have had deep infection. One of these had previously had a septic arthritis and I wonder if there is any connection.

I have seen two fractured ceramic liners, one with an unsupported rim and the other in a man of 146 kilos.

Another obese man has a hip that creaks but is painless.

I have an unbonded HA cup in a revision case where the host bone was not satisfactory for HA fixation. He has buttock pain.

One patient was explored for pain and found to have Pigmented Villo Nodular Synovitis. Two others have unexplained pain but they have had multiple injuries and operations in the past and have never been pain free. Is the pain related to the hip joint?

Whilst I am here I will mention one patient who fractured her ceramic head which was articulating with a plastic liner. The fragments were sent away for examination but no defect in the ceramic was detected. The problem was thought to have arisen as a result of 3 body wear between the spigot and the head.

Conclusions

1. Hydroxyapatite works as a system of implant fixation.
2. Ceramic on Ceramic bearings cannot induce polythene debris disease.
3. Ceramic on Ceramic bearings should be considered where life expectancy is substantial
4. The smooth surface of the bearings should create minimal wear debris.
5. The ceramic material must be properly supported to prevent fracture.
6. The numbers in this series are small and the follow up is short but encouraging.

1.4 Hip HA-Coated Prostheses and Ceramic-on-Ceramic Bearing Surface – A Reliable Solution for Young Patients

J.-P. Vidalain

Introduction

A longer life expectancy, specific pathologies, sternuous professional activities and sometimes the practice of a sport, are the main characteristics of the population in need of a hip arthroplasty before the age of 50.

Many new ideas have been proposed in the past for improving the overall results both in terms of the quality of life and in terms of the lifetime of the arthroplasty components. However, many disappointing clinical outcomes associated with a high rate of mechanical failures, have justified the attitude of only using a total hip replacement once the reasonable limits of a conservative treatment have been passed.

In 1997, the conclusions of the SOFCOT Symposium devoted to THR before 50, demonstrated:
1. The relatively high degree of reliability of total hip prostheses implanted in patients younger than 50, with 85% rate of survival at 10 years,
2. Comparable results in term of survivorship for cemented prostheses and for HA coated prostheses, but with radio-clinical outcomes probably more in favor of bio-active implants (82% of the patients of the HA group are classified as A, only 45% have the same evaluation in the Non-HA group).
3. The recurrent problem of PE wear, whatever the material or the diameter of the prosthetic head.

A personal study presented at the "European Hip Society" in 1998, reporting a continuous series of 131 CORAIL prostheses implanted before 50 years-old, with a mean FU of 6 years, clearly showed that, although the rate of stem survival was 99% at 10 years, the life expectation of the entire arthroplasty unit was only 97% (and 94% for the cup). Moreover, 10% of patients presented radiological modifications slowly evolutive, basically represented by osteolysis related with PE granuloma.

These lesions were observed only in the proximal regions (zones 1 and 7), and never led to mechanical loosening of the shaft. When a revision to change the liner or the cup, has been performed, the different cysts were curetted and grafted with satisfactory results.

The original implant to bone bonding, the absence of fibrous tissue at the interface does actually restrict fluids circulation and particles migration. However, in an ideal situation, it seems logical to keep clear of bearing surfaces generating debris potentially dangerous for the durability of the interface and the stability of the prosthesis.

Material and Methods

Our experience of combination of a "ceramic on ceramic" bearing surface and a HA-coated prosthesis is based on 2 sets of data: the first one, for 47 patients operated on in 1989–1990, and the second one, for 63 prostheses implanted in 1997–1998.

In all cases, the femoral prosthesis was a CORAIL stem. The prosthetic head was either a BIOLOX or a BIOLOX FORTE ceramic ball in 28 mm diameter, and the acetabular component was a press-fit metalbacked shell matched with a ceramic insert provided by the same company. In the first series, an ATOLL cup was used, the convexity of the shell featuring simply a corrundum blasted surface before HA spraying. Nevertheless, several holes allowed the use of additional screws to improve the initial stability. In the second series, the external surface of the cup called LAGOON, presented original macrostructures to increase the mechanical stability, in addition with HA coating treatment. Therefore, a totally blind cup could be used.

Thus, the two series cannot be considered as strictly homogeneous and do not permit overall statistical conclusions to be drawn. However, the quality of the clinical results and above all, the stability in term of radiological issues in the first set, enable us to look forward with optimism the future of patients in the second set. The early functional results satisfy all the requirements of this young population.

There is no need to further comment on the demographical data (age, sex, height and weight), since this simply describes a standard active population. 27% had an arduous profession, 12% wanted to continue participating in a leisure sport. ⅔ of the patients were in Charnley category A.

With all these patients, the operation was a primary implantation justified above all by aseptic necrosis or post-traumatic arthrosis. There was no major dysplasia nor inflammatory arthritis.

Results and Discussion

From a functional point of view, the pains were the main complaint of patients who had ceased their activities several months before (Global pre-operative score: 11.25).

The operation itself presented no difficulty, the stability of the cup was always considered to be good, but in its first version, the addition of radial screws was required 2 out of 3 times, this mechanical problem being solved in the second version.

Full weight bearing has always been allowed immediately and, after a short period of functional rehabilitation, most patients have been able to continue with their previous occupations. 94% of these have been assessed as very satisfactory. The overall score at the last check-up is 17.7; all the hips are more or less pain free, with an improvement in this parameter of 3.2.

There is no specific complications, in particular during the operation. We have not encountered any late complications notably with the bone-prosthesis interface, for either of the components.

X-ray analysis is remarkable for the stability of the pictures and for the "radiological silence" all along the successive check-up:
- Osteointegration of the components, with the production of newly formed bone is evident around the shaft, sometimes also in the region of the dome of the cup in the event of lack of primary contact. The X-ray images are quite identical at each control after the first post-operative year.
- The stability of the implants is perfect; no migration having been detected by conventional radiological techniques.
- The absence of radiolucent lines is characteristic.
- Physiological remodeling is actually limited. At the acetabular level, the bone density is homogeneous, the immediate surroundings of the screws do not exhibit any modification. At the femoral level, there is no sign of stress-shielding apart from a slight remodeling of the calcar. No osteolysis, no cortical reaction, no pedestal.
- With regard to the bearing surfaces, no modification has been assessable during follow-up, specially with the first series of patients.
- None of the ceramic components has fractured.

Conclusions

These findings demonstrate the advantages in an arthroplasty integrating most of the improvements which are recognized as reliable and likely to contribute to the durability of implant fixation in very active patients.

Thus, it seems that the combination of HA-coated prostheses and ceramic on ceramic bearings, can be reasonably proposed to younger patients who are looking for minima restrictions in the quality of life, by reducing the risk of revision as far as possible.

1.5 Why Selecting the Ceramic on Ceramic Bearing Couple?

Ph. Maury, E. Gagneux, F. Gautier, S. Didelot

Why Should We Need to Change the THR Bearing Couple?

Most hip prostheses currently use a wear couple of metal on polyethylene or ceramic on polyethylene with a life span of more than 15 years, sometimes much more, as can be seen in certain Charnley prostheses which are 30 years old. This longevity is suited to patients over 65 years old, but is very insufficient for younger, more active patients.

Furthermore, the longevity of these implants is entirely dependant on the wear of the polyethylene, and more importantly, on the wear debris which accumulate in the periprosthetic vicinity. These particles, as we know, are responsible for the macrophagic reaction, which causes osteolysis and leads to the aseptic loosening of the implant. This debris release is even more extensive if the subject is active [18]. Moreover, there exists a proportional correlation between the number of particles and the extent of osteolysis [1,14].

It is thus imperative to find a wear couple with a low level of particle release, yet is resistant to the stresses brought about by an active, even athletic, life, and which is resistant to shocks.

Two Couples are Currently in Competition: The Ceramic on Ceramic and the Metal on Metal Couples

For the last ten years, research has been carried out principally on these two couples where the wear rate appears to be very low.

The ceramic on ceramic couple

Use of this couple in hip prostheses dates back to 1970–1973. The first series [2,8,10,13,29,31] showed that if the wear rate proved to be less than with PE-metal on ceramic on metal couple, the level of failure remained high. These failures were mainly attributed to the fracture of the ceramic components and premature loosening by periprosthetic osteolysis [14,24,30,32]. Responsibility for the different factors was attributed to the design of the implant (cotyle of Mittelmeier), or the presence of wear debris in the periprosthetic tissues (Zirconia in particular, alumina to a lesser degree), or the faulty positioning of the implants [1, 4].

The 80's saw the introduction of new ceramics with very much improved characteristics, in particular due to the use of alumina powders (Al_2O_3), very pure (99.9%), and low in roughness (0.005 µ). The zirconia on zirconia couple was completely abandoned, the use of this ceramic being currently limited to the combination of a zirconia head articulating against a polyethylene cup (we are only treating alumina ceramics here). The crucial point of the inadequate mechanical resistance of the material, as seen in the high number of implant fractures, was resolved by improvements in the material itself (see Table 1) and by a modification in the design of the prosthetic head [7].

Tests carried out on a simulator with these new ceramics, and the medium-term revisions (10 years), confirmed a low wear rate, 0.003 mm/yr for Skinner [23], 0.016 mm/yr for Jazrawi [12], and 0.025 µ/yr for Dorlot [4]. Similarly, the percentage of prosthetic head fractures

Table 1 Mechanical resistance (o4 p test, from CeramTec)

	MPa
1970	400
1985: Biolox	500
1995: Biolox forte	580

fell to 0.06% for Fritsch [7], and even less than 0.02% for Willmann [26].

The latter author tackled the problem of poor osteo-integration of the ceramic monoblock cotyles [27]. Two concepts are currently proposed: ceramic insert + metal back (type Céralock), or a "sandwich" of a polyethylene layer interposed between the ceramic and metal envelope [28].

The first published series appeared encouraging over a 10-year follow-up. Nizard [17], publishing a series of 187 arthroplasties over a 10-year follow-up, announced a survival rate of 99.16% for the femoral stem, and 88.5% for the acetabular cup. Sedel [19] confirmed these good results with a survival rate of 98% at 10 years for patients younger than 50. Jazrawi [12] reported less good results for loosening at 12 years, but confirmed a wear rate in vivo of 0.016 mm/yr.

The metal on metal couple

This couple was tried very early on with the McKee prosthesis. Its development was marked by some early loosening, characterized by severe osteolysis due to major metallosis. The problem of aseptic loosening brought this experiment to a stop at the end of the 70's. However, the long-term results of some of these prostheses remain a mystery, with a survival rate of sometimes over 30 years, without wear [25]. These cases encouraged some to launch the metal on metal couple.

It is still in the research stage, in the absence of a series with a sufficient time lapse. But the tests in vitro are encouraging, particularly concerning wear rate. Sieber [22] described a phenomenon of "breaking in" with a wear rate of 25 µ/yr the first year, then from the third year, a reduction of this level of 5 µ/yr. Clarke [3] obtained a wear of 0.119 mm³/million cycles, Semlitsch [21] announced 2 to 20 µ/yr.

Which Couple Should We Chose?

The ceramic on ceramic couple seems to us more effective than the metal on metal couple. The results from the in vitro experiments show that the two couples enable a notable reduction in wear debris, but with a greater phenomenon of "breaking in" for the metal one (see Table 2) [1,5,6,22].

The overall volume of particles released into the periprosthetic vicinity appears, therefore, to be much greater in the medium term for metal than for ceramic. Furthermore, the metallic particles generate a histiocytic reaction very quickly (thus osteolytic granulomas), whereas ceramic seems to be practically bioinert [9,11,16]. The lack of a time lapse with regard to metal does not allow us to lift this question, whereas the alumina on alumina couple, over a 10-year follow-up, confirms, so far, the hopes it had aroused.

Table 2 Comparative wearing of metal on metal and ceramic on ceramic couple

Material	Volumetric wear mm³/year per million cycles	
	Initial	Steady state
Metal on metal	0.31	0.03
Ceramic on ceramic	0.12	0.05

after Fisher et al. [6]

Conclusion

To conclude, our choice is guided by a main objective which is the long-term survival of an artificial joint.

The alumina on alumina couple answers, for the moment, to these requirements, as much on the experimental level as on the clinical. The metal on metal couple seems to us a bit less attractive, and must still largely prove itself before competing with ceramic.

References

1. Böhler M, Mochida Y, Bauer ThW, Salzer M (1999) Analysis of wear debris particles from Alumina on Alumina Ceramic THA. In: Reliability and long-term results of ceramics in orthopaedics, Georg Thieme Verlag, Stuttgart: 57–59
2. Boutin P, Christel P, Dorlot JM, Meunier A, de Roquancourt A, Blanquaert D, Herman S, Sedel L, Witvoet J (1988) The use of dense alumina-alumina ceramic combination in total hip replacement. J Biomet Mater Res 22 (12): 1203–32
3. Clarke IC, Anissian L, Stark A, Gustafson A, Good V, Williams P, Downs B, Yu L (1999) Comparisons of M-M and M-PE hip systems at 10 million cycles in hip simulator study. In Metasul: a metal-on-metal bearing, Hans Huber, Berne 93–109

4. Dorlot JM, Christel P, Meunier A (1989) Wear analysis of retrieved alumina heads and sockets of hip prostheses. J Biomet Mater Res 23 (A3 Suppl): 299–310
5. Dorlot JM (1992) Long-term effect of alumina components in total hip prostheses. Clin Orthop 282: 47–52
6. Fisher J, Ingham E, Stone MH, Wroblewski BM, Barbour PSM, Besong AA, Tipper JL, Matthews JB, Firkins PJ, Nevelos AB, Nevelos JE (1999) Wear and debris generation in artificial hip joints. In: Reliability and long-term results of ceramics in orthopaedics, Georg Thieme Verlag, Stuttgart 78–81
7. Fritsch EW, Gleitz M (1996) Ceramic femoral head fractures in total hip arthroplasty. Clin Orthop 328: 129–36
8. Hoffinger SA, Keggi KJ, Zatorski LE (1991) Primary hip replacement: a prospective study of 119 hips. Orthopedics 14 (5): 523–31
9. Huo MH, Salvati EA, Lieberman JR, Betts F, Bansal M (1992) Metallic debris in femoral endosteolysis in failed cemented total hip arthroplasties. Clin Orthop 276: 157–68
10. Huo MH, Martin RP, Zatorski LE, Keggi KJ (1996) Total hip replacement using the ceramic Mittelmeier prosthesis. Clin Orthop (332): 143–50
11. Jacobs JJ, Skipor AK, Patterson LM, Hallab NJ, Paprosky WG, Black J, Galante JO (1998) Metal release in patients who have had a primary total hip arthroplasty. A prospective, controlled, longitudinal study. J Bone Joint Surg Am 80 (10): 1447–58
12. Jazrawi LM, Bogner E, Della Valle CJ, Chen FS, Pak KI, Stuchin SA, Frankel VH, Di Cesare PE (1999) Wear rate of ceramic on ceramic bearing surfaces in total hip implants: a 12-year follow-up study. J Arthoplasty 14 (7): 781–7
13. Kummer FJ, Stuchin SA, Frankel VH (1990) Analysis of removed autophor ceramic on ceramic components. J Arthroplasty 5 (1): 28–33
14. Lerouge S, Huk O, Yahia LH, Sedel L (1996) Characterization of in vivo wear debris from ceramic-ceramic total hip arthroplasties. J Biomed Mater Res 32 (4): 627–33
15. Lerouge S, Huk O, Yahia L, Witvoet J, Sedel L (1997) Ceramic-ceramic and metal-polyethylene total hip replacements: comparison of pseudomembranes after loosening. J Bone Joint Surg Br 79: 135–9
16. Li J, Liu Y, Hermansson L, Soremark R (1993) Evaluation of biocompatibility of various ceramic powders with human fibroblasts in vitro. Clin Mater 12 (4): 197–201
17. Nizard RS, Sedel L, Christel P, Meunier A, Soudry M, Witvoet J (1992) Ten-year survivorship of cemented ceramic-ceramic total hip prosthesis. Clin Orthop 282: 53–63
18. Pappas MJ, Makris G, Buechel FF (1995) Titanium nitride ceramic film against polyethylene. A 48 million cycle wear test. Clin Orthop 317: 64–70
19. Sedel L, Kerboull L, Christel P, Meunier A, Witvoet J (1990) Alumina-on-alumina hip replacement. Results and survivorship in young patients. J Bone Joint Surg Br 72: 658–63
20. Sedel L (1999) Evolution of alumina/alumina implants. In: Reliability and long-term results of ceramics in orthopaedics, Georg Thieme Verlag, Stuttgart 2–6
21. Semlitsch M, Willert HG (1997) Clinical wear behavior of ultra-high molecular weight polyethylene cups paired with metal and ceramic ball heads in comparison to metal-on-metal pairings of hip joint replacement. Proc Inst Mech Eng 211: 73–88
22. Sieber HP, Rieker CB, Kottig P (1999) Analysis of 118 second-generation metal-on-metal retrieved hip implants. J Bone Joint Surg Br 81: 46–50
23. Skinner HB (1999) Ceramic bearing surfaces. Clin Orthop 369: 83–91
24. Toni A, Stea S, Squarzoni S, Sudanese A, Masetti G, Maraldi N, Pizzoferrato A, Giunti A (1992) Considerations on ceramic prosthesis explants. Chir Organi Movi 77 (4): 359–71
25. Weber BG (1999) Metasul from 1988 to today. In Metasul. A metal-on-metal bearing, Hans Huber, Berne 23–28
26. Willmann G, Pfaff HG, Richter HG (1995) Increasing the safety of ceramic femoral heads for hip prostheses. Biomed Tech 40 (12): 342–6
27. Willmann G (1997) Ceramic cups for hip endoprostheses. 3: On the problem of osseointegration of monolithic cups. Biomed Tech 42 (9): 256–63
28. Willmann G, Kramer U (1998) Ceramic cups for hip endoprostheses. 5: Consideration of design. Biomed Tech 43 (12): 342–9
29. Winter M, Griss P, Scheller G, Moser T (1992) Ten- to 14-year results of a ceramic hip prosthesis. Clin Orthop 282: 73–80
30. Wirganowicz PZ, Thomas BJ (1997) Massive osteolysis after ceramic on ceramic total hip arthroplasty. A case report. Clin Orthop 338: 100–4
31. Wu CC, Shih CH (1998) Cementless ceramic total hip arthroplasty: a 5- to 16-year follow-up. Chang Keng I Hsueh Tsa Chih 119: 300–5
32. Yoon TR, Rowe SM, Jung ST, Seon KJ, Maloney WJ (1998) Osteolysis in association with a total hip arthroplasty with ceramic bearing surfaces. J Bone Joint Surg Am 80 (10): 1459–68

1.6 Modular Press-Fit Acetabular Components in Total Hip Arthroplasty

A Comparative Clinical Trial Using Polyethylene and Alumina Liners

R. P. Pitto, D. Schwämmlein, M. Schramm

Abstract

Modular acetabular components with alumina liners are currently used in total hip arthroplasty, but concerns have emerged regarding their high stiffness, which could cause impairment of primary stability, stress-shielding phenomena, and loosening. The purpose of the present investigation was to provide treatment outcome information for total hip arthroplasty patients who received a modular acetabular component inserted with an alumina liner, and to compare the results to those of patients who received the same acetabular component inserted with a polyethylene liner.

Forty-nine consecutive patients (50 hips) with osteoarthrosis scheduled for primary total hip arthroplasty treatment were included in the clinical trial. The first group of 25 hips received a modular press-fit cup with a polyethylene liner and an alumina femoral head. The second group of 25 hips was operated on using the same cup, but an alumina liner was inserted instead of polyethylene. The mean age of patients at index operation was 61 years, and the mean follow-up was 4.5 years (min. 4 years, max. 5 years). Current criteria were used for clinical and radiological assessment.

At the time of the latest follow-up, one patient (one hip, 2%) had been lost, and 2 patients (2 hips, 4%) had died. However, the status of the hip joint at the time of death could be verified in both patients. Thus, the clinical outcome of 48 patients (49 hips, 98%) was known. Radiographs were available for 46 patients (47 hips) who were alive for the entire follow-up period. The mean preoperative Harris hip score was rated 53. At the time of follow-up the mean score has improved to 94. The score was rated good in 30 hips and excellent in 18 hips. One patient (one hip, 2%) had a fair clinical result owing to persisting limp. In the present series no hip required revision, and there was no radiographic evidence of aseptic loosening at follow-up. No sign of cup migration were observed. Radiolucencies without progression were found in the DeLee-Charnely zone 1 in 2 of 47 hips (4.3%), and in the zone 3 in 4 hips (8.5%). No statistically significant differences of results was observed between the two groups of hips.

At an average of 4.5 years postoperatively, the acetabular component inserted with an alumina liner functioned well overall and patient satisfaction was high. Clinical and radiological results do not contrast with those achieved using the same cup with a polyethylene liner.

Introduction

An increasing number of primary total hip arthroplasties are performed in the world with success (18, 30). Contemporary surgical techniques for the insertion of the acetabular and femoral component have been improved and offer a high standard of quality (2,11,19). Nevertheless, wear debris and aseptic loosening still constitutes the major issue and seems greatly dependent to the quality of fixation, implant design and biomaterials (1,6,7,15,22,26).

Previous studies showed a substantial reduction of wear debris using alumina-alumina pairing (13, 29). The modern alumina-alumina pairing requires the use of modular acetabular components (25,31). Recently, concerns have emerged regarding the high stiffness of modular cups with alumina liners, which could cause impairment of primary stability, stress-shielding phenomena, and early loosening (4,23,27).

Assessment of results provides baseline information for refining indications and defining causes of failure. The purpose of the present investigation was to achieve treatment outcome information for total hip arthroplasty patients who

Table 1 Data on the patients. The values are given as the mean and the standard deviation

Parameter	Group 1 (polyethylene) 24 patients (25 hips)	Group 2 (alumina) 25 patients (25 hips)
Gender (M/F)	M = 8; F = 16	M = 10; F = 15
Age (years)	62 ± 4.5	60 ± 5.5
Weight (kg)	70 ± 9	73 ± 8
Height (cm)	172 ± 12	169 ± 9
Fuctional status (Charnley rating)	A = 21 hips B = 4 hips	A = 19 hips B = 6 hips
Duration of operation (mins)	68 ± 8	70 ± 12

received a modular acetabular component inserted with an alumina liner, and to compare the outcome to those of patients who received the same acetabular component with a polyethylene liner.

Material and Methods

Fifty hips (49 patients) operated on between march 1995 and december 1996 were included in a prospective, comparative study. The main criteria for inclusion were primary and secondary osteoarthrosis, quality of the bone adequate for uncemented fixation, and age at index operation less than 70 years. The main criteria for exclusion were rheumatoid arthritis, fracture, and systemic disease directly impairing the act of walking. The mean age of patients at index operation was 61 years (Table **1**).

The indication for total hip arthroplasty was primary coxarthrosis in 38 hips, dysplasia in 7 hips, and avascular necrosis of the femoral head in 5 hips. Two hips has previous operations. Total hip arthroplasty was performed in general anesthesia with the patient placed in the supine position. The hip joint was exposed through the direct lateral approach. A modular acetabular component (Phönix, Brehm, Weisendorf, Germany) (Fig. **1**) was inserted in 25 hips using a polyethylene liner. The same cup was inserted in the remaining 25 hips with an alumina liner (Biolox Forte, CeramTec, Plochingen, Germany). All hips received an alumina femoral head with a diameter of 28 mm (Biolox Forte). An uncemented femoral component was used in 48 hips. In 2 hips the femoral component was cemented. Postoperatively, touch weight bearing up to 20 kg was allowed over the first 6 weeks, then progressively

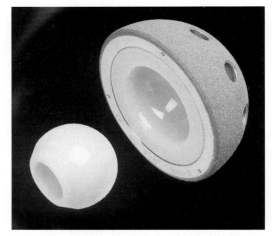

Fig. 1 The Phönix cup is a TiAl6Nb7 modular press-fit acetabular component with a pure-titanium powder coating (TiRC®). The thickness of the coating ranges between 200 and 300 µm, the porosity R_z ranges between 100 and 120 µm. The articular surface liner can be made either of polyethylene or of alumina.

increased loading to full weight bearing within the next 2 weeks. Patients were clinically assessed using the Harris hip score. Evaluation of the femoral and acetabular components was performed using published criteria (14). Radiolucent lines were assessed according to the suggestions of Freeman (9). Location of radiolucent lines, osteolysis and cortical hypertrophy was defined according to the DeLee-Charnley and Gruen criteria (8,10). For evaluation of heterotopic ossification the Brooker classification was used (5). Stress shielding was classified as grade I when only resorption of the medial edge of the resection line appeared. Grade II means additional proximal

Table 2 Radiological findings. The values are given as the mean and the standard deviation

Parameter	Group 1 (polyethylene) 24 patients (25 hips)	Group 2 (alumina) 25 patients (25 hips)
Acetabular angle	40° (±3°)	35° (±4°)
Stability of acetabular cup	bony ingrowth	bony ingrowth
Proximal migration of cup	none	none
Lateral migration of cup	none	none
Tilting of cup	none	none
Radiolucent lines (cup)	DeLee-Charnley zone 1 (1 hip) DeLee-Charnley zone 2 (none) DeLee-Charnley zone 3 (3 hips)	DeLee-Charnley zone 1 (1 hip) DeLee-Charnley zone 2 (none) DeLee-Charnley zone 3 (1 hip)
Axis of femoral stem	neutral (20 hips) valgus (3 hips) varus (2 hips)	neutral (18 hips) valgus (5 hips) varus (2 hips)
Migration of stem	none	none
Radiolucent lines (stem)	Gruen zone 1 (3 hips) Gruen zone 7 (2 hips)	Gruen zone 1 (2 hips) Gruen zone 7 (2 hips)
Heterotopic ossification	Brooker I (3 hips)	Brooker I (2 hips)

medial bone resorption, grade III findings extended more distally (3).

Statistical Analysis

The demographic and radiological data were analyzed with a two-tailed, unpaired t test. A repeated measures analysis of variance and a Newman-Keuls test for intergroup comparisions were performed for all the radiological determination. Multivariate analysis was performed to identify the particular combinations of clinical and radiological findings. Differences were considered statistically significant with the values of $p \leq 0.05$.

Results

There was no significant difference among the two groups of patients in respect to gender, age, body weight, height, function, and joint pathology. Both cemented stems were inserted in the alumina group of hips. At the time of the latest follow-up, one patient (one hip, 2%) had been lost, and 2 patients (2 hips, 4%) had died. However, the status of the hip joint at the time of death could be verified in both patients. Thus, the clinical outcome of 48 patients (49 hips, 98%) was known. Radiographs were available for 46 patients (47 hips) who were alive for the entire 4.5-year follow-up period (4 to 5 years). The mean preoperative Harris hip score was rated 53 (min. 47, max. 69), and it has improved to 94 (min 87, max. 98) at the time of follow-up. The score was good for 30 hips and excellent for 18 hips, so the rate of clinical success was 98%. Occasional pain was present in one hip (2%). Range of joint motion was limited to less than 110° in 3 hips (6%), and 2 patients (2 hips, 4%) were unable to walk without a cane. Dysplasia of the hip joint showed a positive correlation to limited range of motion and function. No difference of clinical results was observed between the two groups of hips.

There was no radiographic evidence of migration or aseptic loosening of the acetabular component at follow-up (Table **2**).

All uncemented acetabular components were considered radiologically stable with complete bone ingrowth (Fig. **2**). Radiolucencies with a periprothetic sclerosis reaction and without progression were found in the DeLee-Charnley zone 1 in 2 of 47 hips (4.3%), and in the zone 3 in 4 hips (8.5%). No radiological signs of wear were detected using conventional measurement methods. No statistically significant difference of radiological results was observed between the two groups of hips.

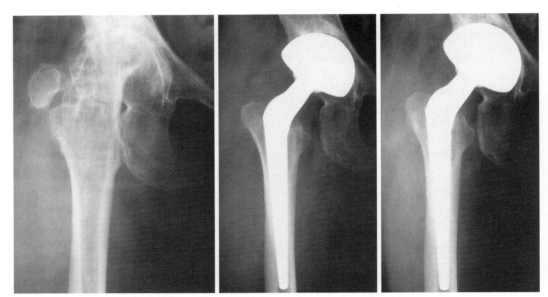

Fig. 2 Anteroposterior radiograph of a 35-year-old woman with severe hip dysplasia and previous operations (left). The postoperative radiograph shows a good alignment of the uncemented prosthesis with an alumina-alumina pairing (centre). There is a radiolucent line in the DeLee-Charnley zone 2, corresponding to a small gap between cup and acetabulum, which was filled using autologous bone grafting. The 4-year follow-up radiograph shows integration of the prosthesis without signs of migration (right). The bone stock is excellent. The Harris hip score is rated 95.

There was no radiographic evidence of migration or aseptic loosening of the femoral component at follow-up. Radiolucencies with a sclerosis reaction at the bone-implant interface without progression were found in the zone 1 in 2 of 47 hips (4.3%), and in the zone 7 in 4 hips (8.5%). Radiolucencies without sclerosis were not detected. A slight cortical hypertrophy was seen in 4 hips (8.5%). thirty-nine of 47 hips (83%) had either no change in femoral bone density or only patchy loss of bone density isolated to Gruen zone 1 and 7. Eight hips (17%) had some reduction of bone density isolated to zone 1 and 7. Heterotopic ossifications were observed in 5 hips (10.6%). Radiological signs of stress shielding rated grade I, with resorption of the medial edge of the resection line, were observed in 41 hips (87%). Bone resorption in the proximal portion of the femur (Gruen zones 1 and 7) which was interpreted as grade II stress shielding was present in the remaining 6 hips (13%). Distal extension of osteolysis into Gruen zones 2 and 6 was not observed. No statistically significant difference of radiological results was observed between the two groups of hips.

Discussion

Polyethylene acetabular liners and alumina femoral heads represent nowadays the standard for total hip arthroplasty treatment (2,18,19). The application is based on the good tribological properties of these materials. An even better tribological combination is represented by an alumina liner and an alumina femoral head (13,31). Alumina on alumina bearings have potential for markedly reducing the volume of particulate wear debris and thereby reducing the loosening that results from osteolysis. Nevertheless, the clinical results of acetabular components inserted with an alumina liner remains controversial (4, 12, 29). Insertion of alumina on alumina bearings requires the use of modular acetabular component with a high modulus of elasticity, and therefore high stiffness. In-vitro analysis showed a 50 times higher stiffness of modular cups with alumina liner compared to identical cups with polyethylene liner (4). This condition could cause unfavourable contact stresses around the periacetabular bone, leading to bone resorption and loosening. Nevertheless, finite-element analysis demontrated a distribution of load approaching the physiological behaviours in cups with alumina liner (12). Furthermore, a biomechanical in-vitro study showed no positive correlation between stiffness and initial stability pattern of modular acetabular components with different design (24, 26).

The specific aims of the present comparative investigation were to assess prospectively the clinical and radiological results of patients operated on using a modular acetabular component with an alumina liner or with a polyethylene liner, in order to provide treatment outcome information and to identify risk factors for poor results. No acetabular component required revision, and there was no difference of outcome in the two study groups. All implants were radiologically stable, with an average Harris hip score of 94 at a mean 4.5-years follow-up. Persistent thigh pain requiring pharmacological or physical treatment was not observed in any of the patients. This finding does not contrast with data reported by other authors using modular acetabular components (13, 29).

The strength of the present paper is represented by the prospective design and by the homogeneous distribution of the patient population into the two study groups. Furthermore, all hips were operated on by a single surgeon. This factor eliminates the effect of the potentially confounding variable of multiple surgeons (14).

The most important limitation of the present study is determined by the short follow-up observation. Early clinical assessment of the performance of a new design of total hip arthroplasty is notoriously unreliable. Full evaluation of outcomes requires a clinical trial of at least 10 years (20). The second limitation of the present study was the conventional technique of radiological assessment. Measurements on conventional radiographs can have an accuracy of 1–5 mm and 1–6° depending on technique employed, the anatomic region investigated, and the number of examiners (21). A method of predicting implant performance as soon as possible after operation is needed, and radiostereoanalysis has this potential (28). It has been shown that radiostereoanalysis can detect abnormalities before there are clinical signs of loosening, and that there is a good correlation between increased migration rate and early loosening (16). Radiostereoanalysis is based on radiographic examinations of calibration cages and object markers implanted in the skeleton. Accurate measurement of radiographs and computer-assisted calculation can provide a three-dimensional motion analysis. Radiostereoanalysis can be performed with an accuracy of 10–250 µm and 0.03–0.6° (17, 28). Owing to the high-accuracy measurements of skeletal movements, radiostereoanalysis represents one of the most reliable methods to perform clinical trials in total hip arthroplasty (Fig. 3). Therefore, we have recently entertained a prospective radiostereoanalysis study in order to determine in-vivo the three-dimensional migration pattern of the Phönix modular cup (Fig. 4). The hips are randomly allocated for treatment with an alumina acetabular liner, or a polyethylene acetabular liner. All hips receive an alumina femoral head with a diameter of 28 mm. The preliminary results show no significant difference of migration pattern in the two study groups.

In conclusion, at an average of 4.5 years postoperatively, the modular acetabular component inserted using an alumina liner functioned well overall and patient satisfaction was high. Clinical and radiological results do not contrast with those achieved using the same cup inserted with a polyethylene liner.

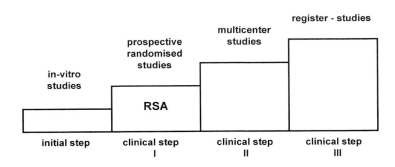

Fig. 3 The fundamental steps for the introduction of a new prosthesis to the market place. Radiostereoanalysis (RSA) plays an important role during the initial clinical trials, and can avoid disastrous experiences on a large scale of patients.

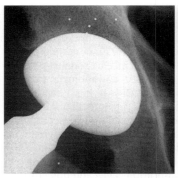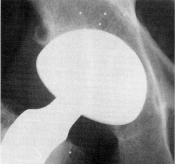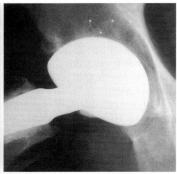

Fig. 4 Postoperative anteroposterior radiograph of a 54-year-old man with primary osteoarthrosis after hybrid total hip arthroplasty using an alumina-alumina pairing (left). Tantalum markers with a diameter of 0.8 mm have been placed in the bone in order to perform radiostereoanalysis. The 2-year anteroposterior and lateral follow-up radiographs show a stable prosthesis without lucent lines (right). There are no signs of migration and the bone stock is excellent. The Harris hip score is rated 98.

References

1. Amstutz HC, Markolf KL, McNeice GM, Gruen TA (1976) Loosening of total hip components: cause and prevention. In: The hip: Proceedings of the fourth open scientific meeting of The Hip Society. C. V. Mosby, St Louis 102–116
2. Berger RA, Kull LR, Rosenberg AG, Galante JO (1996) Hybrid total hip arthroplasty. Clin Orthop 333: 134–145
3. Bobyn JD, Mortimer ES, Glassman A (1992) Producing and avoiding stress shielding. Laboratory and clinical observations of noncemented total hip arthroplasty. Clin Orthop 274: 79–96
4. Boehler M, Krismer M, Mayr G, Muehlbauer M, Salzer M (1998) Migration measurement of cementless acetabular components: value of clinical and radiographic data. Orthopaedics 21: 897–900
5. Brooker AE, Bowerman JW, Robinson RA, Riley LH (1973) Ectopic ossification following total hip replacement. Incidence and a method of classification. J Bone Joint Surg 55-A: 1629–1632
6. Charnley J (1979) Low friction arthroplasty of the hip. Springer-Verlag, Berlin Heidelberg New York
7. Coventry MB (1992) Lessons lerned in 30 years of total hip arthroplasty. Clin Orthop 274: 22–29
8. DeLee J, Charnley J (1976) Radiological demarcation of cemented sockets in total hip replacement. Clin Orthop 121: 20–30
9. Freeman MAR (1999) Radiolucent lines. A question of nomenclature. J Arthroplasty 14: 1–2
10. Gruen TA, McNeice GM, Amstutz HC (1979) Mode of failure of cemented stem-type femoral components: a radiographic analysis of loosening. Clin Orthop 141: 17–27
11. Harris WH, McGann WA (1982) Loosening of the femoral component after use of medullary plug cement technique. J Bone Joint Surg 64-A: 1063–1067
12. Hendrich C, Kaddick C, Willmann G (1999) Krafteinleitung in das knöcherne Becken bei keramischen Pfanneneinsätzen. Eine Finite-Elemente-Analyse. Z Orthop 137, A31
13. Heros R, Willmann G (1998) Ceramics in total hip arthroplasty. Seminars in Arthroplasty 9: 114–122
14. Johnston RC, Fitzgerald RH, Harris WH, Poss R, Müller ME, Sledge CB (1990) Clinical and radiological evaluation of total hip replacement. J Bone Joint Surg 72-A: 1025–1034
15. Joshi RP, Eftekhar NS, McMahon DJ, Nercessian OA (1998) Osteolysis after Charnley primary low-friction arthroplasty. J Bone Joint Surg 80-B: 585–590
16. Kärrholm J (1997) Radiostereometry of hip prostheses. Clin Orthop 344: 94–110
17. Kiss J, Murray DW, Turner-Smith AR, Bithell J, Bulstrode CJ (1996) Migration of cemented femoral components after total hip replacement. J Bone Joint Surg 78-B: 796–801
18. Malchau H, Herberts P (1998) Prognosis of total hip replacement. Revision and re-revision rate in THR: A revision-risk study of 148,359 primary operations. The national hip arthroplasty registry. Scientific exhibition presented at the 65th annual meeting of the American Academy of Orthopaedic surgeons. February, New Orleans, USA
19. Mulroy WF, Estok DM, Harris WH (1995) Total hip arthroplasty with use of so-called second-generation cementing techniques. J Bone Joint Surg 77-A: 1845–1852

20 Murray DW (1999) Outcome studies of hip replacement. Instructional course lectures of the European Federation of National Associations of Orthopaedics and Traumatology 4: 83–87
21 Nunn D, Freeman MAR, Hill PF, Evans SJW (1989) The measurement of migration of the acetabular component of hip prostheses. J Bone Joint Surg 71-B: 629–631
22 Pitto RP, Sterzl M (1995) Acetabular Micromotion as a Measure of the Initial Stability of a Press-Fit Implant. Transactions of the 5th EORS Annual Conference 135
23 Pitto RP (1996) Evaluation of acetabular initial micromotion in press-fit cups. International Orthopaedics 20: 396
24 Pitto RP, Sterzl M, Hohmann D (1996) Observations on the initial stability of acetabular components in total hip arthroplasty. An experimental study. Chir Organi Mov. 81: 107–118
25 Pitto RP (1997) Biomechanical and tribological aspects of press-fit acetabular components. Cera-News 6: 3–4
26 Pitto RP, Böhner J, Hofmeister V (1997) Einflußgrößen der Primärstabilität acetabulärer Komponenten. Eine in-vitro Studie. Biom Technik 42: 363–368
27 Schneider E, Schönenberger U, Giraud P, Bürgi M (1992) Primärstabilität und Beckendeformation bei zementierten und nichtzementierten Hüftpfannen. Orthopäde 21: 57–62
28 Schwämmlein D, Spath A, Opitz U, Pitto RP (1999) Röntgenstereometrische Analyse – ein dreidimensionales Meßverfahren zur Erkennung von Mikrobewegungen der Prothese im totalen Hüftgelenkersatz. Orthopädische Praxis 35: 440–442
29 Sedel L (1999) Tribology and clinical experience of alumina-alumina articulations. Proceedings of the 66th Annual Meeting of the American Academy of Orthopaedic Surgeons 120
30 Stringa G, Di Muria GV, Marcucci M, Pitto RP (1991) Long term results of Charnley low-friction arthroplasty: A thirteen-year average follow-up study. Hip International 1: 21–25
31 Willmann G, Kramer U (1998) Keramische Pfannen für Hüftendoprothesen. Konzeptionelle Überlegungen. Biom Tech 43: 342–349

1.7 Klinische Erfahrungen und Migrationsanalyse – PLASMACUP

C. Hendrich, M. Blanke, U. Sauer, C. P. Rader, J. Eulert

Zusammenfassung

Neue modulare Pfannenkonzepte erlauben neben der Verwendung des Polyäthylen-(PE)-Inlays auch den Einsatz von keramischen Pfanneneinsätzen. Auf Grund der höheren Steifigkeit der Keramik ist eine geänderte Lastübertragung in das knöcherne Implantatlager anzunehmen. So konnte in einer Finite Elemente-Analyse bei Verwendung des Keramik-Inlays eine breitere Lastübertragung in der Peripherie des Implantates simuliert werden. Ziel der vorliegenden Studie war es, anhand einer röntgenologischen Migrationsanalyse den Einfluss der durch das Keramikinlay geänderten Lastübertragung klinisch zu überprüfen.

Im Rahmen einer multizentrischen prospektiv-randomisierten Studie wurden von 1997– 1999 in unserer Klinik 80 Patienten unter 65 Jahren mit PLASMACUP-Pfannen und BiCONTACT-Schäften (Aesculap AG, Tuttlingen) zementfrei versorgt. Jeweils die Hälfte der Patienten erhielten PE- bzw. Keramik-Einsätze. 25 Patienten mit beiden Gleitpaarungen wurden über 2 Jahre regelmäßig klinisch und radiologisch untersucht. Die Diagnosen waren primäre Coxarthrose (n = 38), Dysplasiecoxarthrose (n = 4), Hüftkopfnekrose (n = 5) und sonstige (n = 1). Das mittlere Alter bei Implantation lag bei 54 ± 7 Jahren. Es handelte sich um 28 Männer und 22 Frauen. Neben der klinischen Untersuchung wurde eine röntgenologische Messung der Pfannenmigration mit Hilfe der Einbildröntgenanalyse (EBRA) durchgeführt.

Innerhalb des Beobachtungszeitraumes wurden 3 Implantate revidiert. In einem Fall kam es zu einem Randabbruch des Keramikinlays, bei einer weiteren Patientin lag eine subprothetische Fraktur nach adäquatem Trauma vor. Bei einem dritten Patienten wurden ausgeprägte heterotope Ossifikationen entfernt. Weitere implantatspezifische Komplikationen waren nicht zu verzeichnen. Die mittlere Beugung betrug 105 ± 21°, der mittlere Harris-Score lag bei 87 ± 13 Punkten. Mit einer Ausnahme waren alle Patienten mit dem Operationsergebnis zufrieden. Bei der röntgenologischen Analyse zeigte sich in der Keramik-Gruppe jeweils einmal ein Lysesaum von unter 1 mm in der Zone I und in der Zone II. In der PE-Gruppe zeigten sich Lysesäume von unter 1 mm in der Zone I einmal, in der Zone II zweimal, in der Zone III zweimal und einmal in der Zone IV. Von 50 Patienten mit ausreichender Bildanzahl waren 46 Patienten mit Hilfe der EBRA auswertbar. 45 Patienten lagen innerhalb der Messgenauigkeit von 1 mm, ein Patient mit einem PE-Inlay zeigte eine Migration 1,7 mm nach kranial. Die mittlere Migration aller Implantate zeigte in der Keramik-Gruppe einen Mittelwert von – 0,16 ± 0,55 mm, in der PE-Gruppe 0,22 ± 0,49 mm. Im t–Test auf Mittelwertgleichheit besteht ein signifikanter Unterschied (p < 0,02). Bei der horizontalen Migration zeigte sich ein Mittelwert von 0,02 ± 0,47 mm in der Keramik-Gruppe, bei den PE-Inlays lag der Mittelwert bei – 0,12 ± 0,53 mm. Der Unterschied ist nicht signifikant (p < 0,35).

Mit Ausnahme des Randabbruchs zeigten sich keine implantatspezifischen Komplikationen. Angesichts des jungen Patientenkollektivs sind die klinischen Resultate als günstig zu betrachten. Bei der röntgenologischen Analyse zeigt sich innerhalb der Beobachtungszeit keine nennenswerte Saumbildung, innerhalb von 2 Jahren ist nur ein Implantat gewandert. Ob die durchschnittlich höhere Kranialmigration der PE-Gruppe auch im Gesamtkollektiv nachweisbar ist und eine klinische Signifikanz hat, bleibt über einen längeren Beobachtungszeitraum zu verfolgen.

Schlüsselwörter: Modulare Pfanneneinsätze, Keramik-Gleitpaarung, klinische Resultate, Migrationsanalyse

Einleitung

Die Implantation der Hüfttotalendoprothese ist eine der erfolgreichsten Operationen überhaupt. Auf Grund der gestiegenen Lebenserwartung stellt die aseptische Lockerung trotz der erheblichen Fortschritte innerhalb der letzten Jahrzehnte weiterhin das zentrale Problem der modernen Hüftendoprothetik dar (4). Als wesentliche Lockerungsursache der Pfannenkomponente wurde die abriebinduzierte Osteolyse identifiziert (16). Im Vergleich zu PE-Komponenten zeigt eine Keramik-Keramik-Gleitpaarung einen um mehrere Größenordnungen geringeren Verschleiß (19). In der ersten Generation der Keramik-Keramik-Gleitpaarung wurden ausschließlich monolitische Pfannen eingesetzt, die im Langzeitverlauf hohe Lockerungsraten aufweisen (2, 7, 13). Als Ursache des Versagens werden ungenügende Materialeigenschaften (20), das Schraubpfannendesign (7), die mangelnde Porosität der knochenseitigen Implantatoberfläche und die hohe Implantatsteifigkeit angegeben (3). Bezüglich der knöchernen Verankerung hat sich in den 90er Jahren die mittel- und langfristige Überlegenheit hemisphärischer Pressfit-Pfannen gezeigt (17). Durch die Verwendung einer Konusklemmung als Inlayverankerung erlauben moderne Pfannendesigns die alternative Verwendung von Pfanneneinsätzen aus Aluminoxid-Keramik, um die optimale Osseointegration der hemisphärischen Pressfit-Pfanne mit den überlegenen Abriebeigenschaften der Keramik zu kombinieren. Durch die Verwendung des keramischen Pfanneneinsatzes wird das gesamte Pfannenimplantat jedoch steifer. Während bei einem PE-Inlay die Steifigkeit durch die Metallkomponente bestimmt wird, kehren sich diese Verhältnisse bei dem Keramik-Einsatz um (1). In Relation zur gesamten Extremität kann der der Einfluss des Keramik-Inlays auf die Dämpfungseigenschaften vernachlässigt werden. Dagegen kann die höhere Steifigkeit des Keramik-Inlays zu einer veränderten Lastübertragung in das knöcherne Acetabulum führen (6). Während die Finite Elemente-Simulation mit dem PE-Inlay eine Konzentration der Energiedichte am Pol des Implantats zeigt, erfolgt die Lastübertragung bei Verwendung des Keramik-Einsatzes vermehrt über die Peripherie der Hemisphäre. Obwohl diese Form der Lastübertragung den natürlichen Verhältnissen näher kommt (12, 18), kann eine klinische Signifikanz aus diesen theoretischen Überlegungen zunächst nicht abgeleitet werden. Um diese Fragestellung zu beantworten, wurde eine multizentrische, prospektiv-randomisierte Studie mit alternativer Verwendung von PE- oder Keramik-Pfanneneinsätzen begonnen. Neben der klinischen und konventionell-radiologischen Untersuchung liegt ein besonderer Schwerpunkt der Studie bei der röntgenologischen Messung der Implantatmigration mit Hilfe des Verfahrens der Einbildröntgenanalyse (EBRA) (10). Im folgenden werden die Zweijahresergebnisse der ersten 50 Patienten dargestellt.

Patienten, Material und Methoden

Studiendesign

An der prospektiv-randomisierten Multicenterstudie nehmen die Klinik für Unfall- und Wiederherstellungschirurgie im Lukaskrankenhaus Bünde, die Berufsgenossenschaftliche Unfallklinik Tübingen und die Orthopädische Universitätsklinik Würzburg teil. Einschlusskriterien waren das Vorliegen einer Arthrose ohne signifikante Knochenerkrankung sowie ein Alter zwischen 35 und 70 Jahren. Alle Patienten erhielten eine PLASMACUP-Pfanne in Kombination mit einem zementfreien BiCONTACT-Prothesenschaft. Jeweils die Hälfte der Patienten wurde mit einem PE- bzw. Keramik-Inlay versorgt.

Würzburger Kollektiv

In unserer Klinik wurden 80 Patienten der Jahre 1997–1999 in die Studie eingeschlossen. Die folgende Auswertung bezieht sich auf die ersten 50 Patienten, die jeweils zur Hälfte mit einem PE- bzw. ein Keramik-Inlay versorgt wurden. Es handelte sich um 28 Männer und 22 Frauen. Das mittlere Alter der Patienten lag bei 54 ± 7 Jahren. Die Diagnosen waren primäre Arthrose (n = 38), Dysplasiecoxarthrose (n = 4), Hüftkopfnekrose (n = 5) sowie eine posttraumatische Coxarthrose (Abb. 1).

Operationsverfahren und Nachuntersuchung

Alle Patienten wurden in Rückenlage operiert. Standardmäßig wurde ein transglutealer Zugang nach Bauer verwendet. Das Aufbereiten des Pfannengrundes erfolgte mit den entsprechenden Raffelfräsen, regelmäßig wurde eine autologe Spongiosaplastik im Pfannengrund verwendet. Bei zwei Implantaten wurde keine zusätzliche

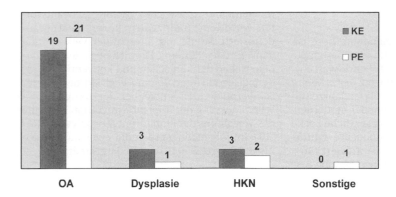

Abb. 1 Verteilung der Diagnosen bei 25 Patienten mit Keramik-Inlay (KE) und 25 Patienten mit Polyäthylen-Inlay (PE).
OA = primäre Coxarthrose, HKN = Hüftkopfnekrose.

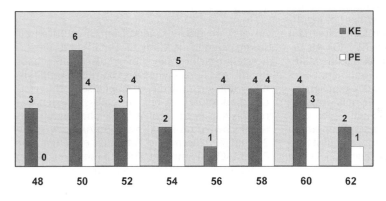

Abb. 2 Pfannengröße bei 25 Patienten mit Keramik-Inlay (KE) und 25 Patienten mit Polyäthyleninlay (PE). Auf der Abszisse sind die verwendeten Implantatgrößen angegeben.

Schraubenfixation verwendet, bei zwei Implantaten eine Schraube, bei 45 Implantaten zwei Schrauben und bei einem Implantat 3 Schrauben. Die Verteilung der Implantatgrößen zeigt Abb. 2. Die Mobilisierung erfolgte am 1. postoperativen Tag. Für insgesamt 6 Wochen wurde eine 20 kg-Teilbelastung erlaubt. Die Röntgenkontrollen erfolgten unmittelbar postoperativ, 14 Tage postoperativ sowie bei regulären Nachuntersuchungen nach 3, 12 und 24 Monaten. Anlässlich der Nachuntersuchung wurde eine ausführliche Anamnese erhoben und eine vollständige orthopädische Untersuchung durchgeführt. Die Röntgenuntersuchung der Beckenübersicht erfolgte liegend mit 10° innenrotiertem Oberschenkel sowie in einer Projektion nach Lauenstein. Die Auswertung der Ergebnisse erfolgte gemäß den Kriterien der Consensus-Study-Group (9). Zur numerischen Darstellung der Resultate wurde der Score nach Harris verwendet.

Einbildröntgenanalyse (EBRA)

Das Verfahren der EBRA wurde erstmals 1988 von einer Arbeitsgruppe der Universität Innsbruck publiziert (15). Das Prinzip beruht auf dem geometrischen Vergleich eines Paßpunktsystems des Beckens mit der Pfannen- und Kopfkontur im Zeitverlauf durch einen sogenannten Vergleichbarkeitsalgorithmus. Zur Durchführung der Messung wird die horizontale Orientierung des Beckens durch Tangenten an der Unterkante des ersten gleichseitigen Foramen sacrale, an den unteren Begrenzungen der Foramina obturatoria und an der Oberkante des Os pubis festgelegt. Die vertikale Orientierung des Beckens werden durch Tangenten an den vertikalen Begrenzungen des Diameter transversum und eine weitere Tangente an der medialen Begrenzung des gleichseitigen Foramen obtoratorium bestimmt. Für die vorliegenden Messungen wurden Röntgenbilder mit einer Schwankungsbreite von 6° in y-Richtung und 3° in x-Richtung zugelassen. Die standardmäßig angefertigten Beckenübersichten

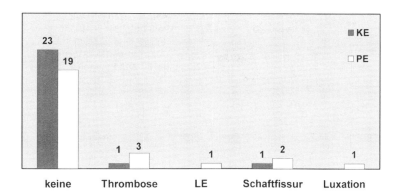

Abb. 3 Komplikationen bei 50 Patienten mit PLASMACUP und BiCONTACT-Schaft. LE = Lungenembolie.

wurden mit einem 10 Bit-Durchlichtscanner (PACE-Systems, Freiburg) digitalisiert und im TIFF-Format gespeichert. Das Anlegen des Tangentensystems erfolgte im Programm EBRA-Digital, Version 1998 (Institut für Geometrie der Universität Innsbruck, Österreich). Die Koordinaten von Beckenkopf und Pfanne werden vom Programm gespeichert, die weiteren Eingaben von Röntgenbildern des selben Patienten werden mit der bestehenden Eingabe verglichen. Die Auswertung einer Messung ist ab einer Mindestanzahl von 4 Bildern pro Patient möglich. Durch den Vergleichbarkeitsalgorithmus, ein Programmmodul, das die Vergleichbarkeit der Röntgenprojektion sicherstellt, wird die Eingabe ungeeigneter Projektionen nicht akzeptiert. Die Darstellung der numerischen Ergebnisse der Pfannenwanderung in x- und y-Richtung im Zeitverlauf und die schematische Darstellung der Wanderung erfolgt als Wanderungstabelle und als entsprechendes Diagramm. Für die Auswertung wurde eine Vergleichbarkeitsschranke von 3 festgelegt, was einer Messgenauigkeit von 1 mm entspricht (8).

Ergebnisse

Perioperative Komplikationen

43 Patienten zeigten keine perioperativen Komplikationen. In 4 Fällen wurde eine Thrombose, einmal mit einer konsekutiven Lungenembolie beobachtet. Schaftfissuren bei 3 Patienten verheilten nach Sicherung mit Drahtzerklagen komplikationslos verheilten. Bei einem Patienten kam es einmalig postoperativ zu einer Luxation. Die Verteilung der perioperativen Komplikationen auf die Keramik- und PE-Gruppe zeigt Abb. **3**.

Revisionen

Drei Patienten wurden innerhalb des Beobachtungszeitraumes erneut operiert. Bei einem 56-jährigen Patienten mit Coxarthrose links erfolgte die Erstimplantation mit Verwendung eines Keramik-Inlays. Anlässlich einer vorgezogenen 12-Monatskontrolle wurde ein Randabbruch des Inlays festgestellt, so dass ein Inlay- und Kopfwechsel erforderlich wurde. Die definitive Schadensanalyse des Inlays steht zur Zeit noch aus.

Eine zweite Patientin wurde im Alter von 48 Jahren bei einer Dysplasiecoxarthrose li. mit einem PE-Inlay versorgt. Nach adäquatem Trauma kam es zu einer subprothetischen Fraktur, die durch Schaftwechsel auf ein modulares Revisionssystem behandelt wurde.

Ein dritter Patient wurde im Alter von 61 Jahren bei Coxarthrose links mit einem Keramik-Inlay versorgt. Trotz Prophylaxe mit Indometacin 2 × 50 mg über 14 Tage wurde bei heterotopen Ossifikationen vom Grad III nach Brooker eine Revision erforderlich.

Anamnese und klinische Untersuchung

20 Patienten verspürten überhaupt keine Schmerzen mehr, 18 Patienten gelegentlich leichte Schmerzen. 8 Patienten gaben mäßige Schmerzen an, während 3 Patienten über einen starken und ein Patient über einen sehr starken Schmerz klagten. Die Verteilung der geklagten Schmerzen war unabhängig von dem verwendeten Inlay. Bei der Untersuchung der Beweglichkeit zeigte sich eine mittlere Flexion von 105 ± 21°, eine Extension von 2 ± 6°, eine Abduktion von 30 ± 7°, eine Adduktion von 21 ± 8°, sowie eine Außenrotation von 30 ± 12° und eine Innenrotation von 22 ± 11°.

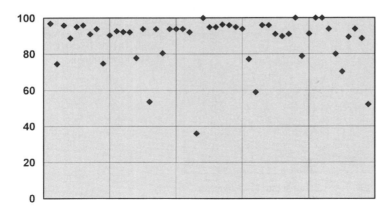

Abb. 4 Harris-Score bei 50 Patienten mit PLASMACUP und BiCONTACT-Schaft. Der mittlere Harris-Score liegt bei 87 ± 13 Punkten.

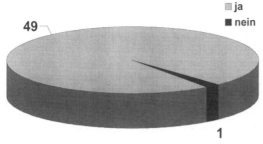

Abb. 5 Zufriedenheit bei 50 Patienten mit PLASMACUP und BiCONTACT-Schaft.

Der kumulierte Harris-Score aller Implantate betrug 87 ± 13 Punkte (Abb. **4**). Während die Keramikgruppe durchschnittlich 89 Punkte aufwies, ergab sich für die PE-Gruppe ein mittlerer Score von 85. Dieser Unterschied war jedoch nicht signifikant. 49 der 50 Patienten waren zufrieden und würden die Operation erneut durchführen lassen, 1 Patient war mit dem Ergebnis unzufrieden (Abb. **5**).

Röntgenbeurteilung

Als Inklinationswinkel waren in der Keramik-Gruppe ein Mittelwert von 35 ± 7° und in der PE-Gruppe von 37 ± 6° zu verzeichnen. Die röntgenologische Messung der Beinlängendifferenz zeigte einmal eine Beinverkürzung von 1,5 cm, bei drei Implantaten einen Unterschied von 1 cm, bei 12 Implantaten von 0,5 cm und bei 34 Patienten ausgeglichene Beinlängen. Alle Pfannenimplantate waren unversehrt, ein Schraubenbruch oder Lysesäume um die Schrauben nicht zu verzeichnen. In der Keramik-Gruppe zeigte je ein Implantat eine Saumbildung von unter 1 mm in der Zone I bzw. in der Zone II. In der PE-Gruppe waren Säume unter 1 mm einmal in der Zone I, zweimal in der Zone II, zweimal in der Zone III und einmal in der Zone IV zu verzeichnen. Eine durchgehende Saumbildung lag in keinem Fall vor.

Einbildröntgenanalyse (EBRA)

Die EBRA ließ sich bei 46 von 50 Implantaten sinnvoll auswerten. Je 2 Implantate der Keramik- und PE-Gruppe waren nicht auswertbar. Bei 45 Implantaten lagen die Messwerte im Bereich der Messgenauigkeit von 1 mm, ein Implantat war über 1 mm gewandert (Abb. **6**). Röntgenverlauf und Wanderungsdiagramm des Patienten sind in Abb. **7** dargestellt. Bei diesem Patienten mit einem PE-Inlay ist es zu einer Kranialisierung von 1,7 mm gekommen. Bei der Analyse der Messwerte aller Implantate zeigt sich für die horizontale Wanderung in der Keramik-Gruppe ein Mittelwert von 0,02 ± 0,47 mm, in der PE-Gruppe von – 0,12 ± 0,53 mm (Abb. **8**). Dieser Unterschied ist im t-Test auf Mittelwertgleichheit nicht signifikant ($p < 0,35$). Die mittlere Kranialmigration liegt bei den Keramikinlays bei – 0,16 ± 0,55 mm, in der PE-Gruppe sind 0,22 ± 0,49 mm zu verzeichnen (Abb. **9**). Im t-Test auf Mittelwertgleichheit ist dieser Unterschied signifikant ($p < 0,02$).

Diskussion

Neue modulare Pfannenkonzepte erlauben eine intraoperative Wahlmöglichkeit der Gleitpaarung. Im Vergleich zum konventionellen PE-Inlay

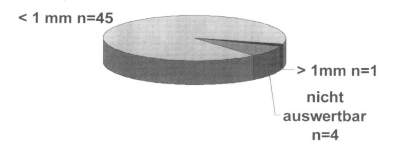

Abb. 6 Einbildröntgenanalyse (EBRA) von 50 Implantaten. 45 Patienten lagen innerhalb des Messbereichs von 1 mm. Ein Patient zeigte eine kraniale Migration von 1,7 mm. Je 2 Patienten aus der Keramik- bzw. Polyäthylen-Gruppe waren nicht auswertbar.

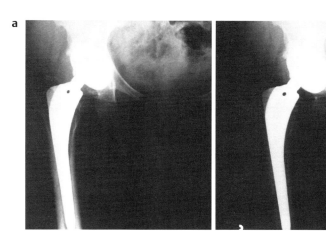

Abb. 7 Röntgenverlauf (**a**) und Migrationsdiagramm (**b**) eines Patienten mit Polyäthylen-Inlay. Dargestellt ist die kraniale Migration von 1,7 mm.

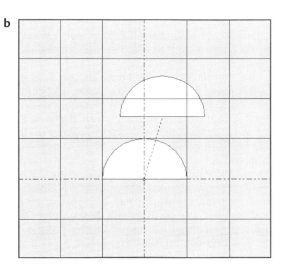

weist das Keramik-Inlay eine wesentlich höhere Implantatsteifigkeit auf. Während der Effekt auf die Dämpfung der gesamten Extremität zu vernachlässigen ist (1), kann nach einer von uns durchgeführten Finite Elemente-Simulation eine geänderte Lastübertragung in das knöcherne Acetabulum angenommen werden (6). Ziel der vorliegenden Studie war die klinische Überprüfung der modularen Pfanneneinsätze im Rahmen einer prospektiv-randomisierten Multicenter-Studie. Neben der klinischen und konventionell-radiologischen Beurteilung sollte vor allem eine Messung der Implantatmigration mit der Einbildröntgenanalyse erfolgen.

Als generelle Einschränkung der Aussagefähigkeit der vorliegenden Studie ist anzuführen, dass es sich nur um ein Teilkollektiv der Gesamtstudie handelt und dass auf Grund der kurzen Beobachtungszeit von 2 Jahren nur eine begrenzte Aussage möglich ist. Andererseits erlaubt gerade die EBRA bereits nach 2 Jahren eine Prognose der Langzeitstabilität. Implantate, die innerhalb der ersten beiden Jahre eine Migration von über

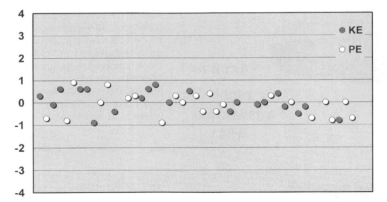

Abb. 8 Horizontale Migration in [mm] von 25 Patienten mit Keramik-Inlay (KE) und 25 Patienten mit Polyäthylen-Inlay (PE). Alle Implantate liegen innerhalb des Messbereichs von 1 mm.

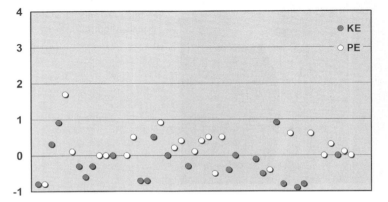

Abb. 9 Kraniale Migration von 25 Patienten mit Keramik-Inlay (KE) und 25 Patienten mit Polyäthylen-Inlay (PE) in [mm]. Während ein Implantat eine kraniale Migration von 1,7 mm aufweist, liegen alle übrigen Pfannen innerhalb des Messbereichs von 1 mm.

1 mm aufweisen, zeigen im Gegensatz zu nicht gewanderten Implantaten eine signifikant höhere Lockerungsrate (11).

Perioperativ zeigen sich für das Pfannenimplantat und insbesondere für den Keramik-Einsatz keine implantatspezifischen Komplikationen. Das Instrumentarium weist keine wesentlichen Schwächen auf. Im Schaftbereich wurde das bewährte BiCONTACT-Implantat verwendet. Die im Kollektiv aufgetretenen Schaftfissuren stellen mittelfristig keine Beeinträchtigung für den Patienten dar. Insgesamt ist die Komplikationsrate als niedrig anzusehen.

Innerhalb des Beobachtungszeitraums wurden 3 Revisionen erforderlich. Hier ist es in einem Fall zu einem Abbruch des Inlayrands gekommen, der durch Inlay- und Kopfwechel behandelt wurden. Die beiden anderen Revisionen sind dagegen nicht implantatspezifisch bedingt. Die endgültige Schadensanalyse des abgebrochenen Inlayrandes steht zum Zeitpunkt dieser Publikation noch aus. Möglicherweise ist es bei diesem Patienten mit einer Beugefähigkeit von 130° zu einem Impingement des Prothesenhalses gekommen.

Bei der Bewertung der klinischen Ergebnisse ist das junge Patientenkollektiv zu berücksichtigen. Im Vergleich zu anderen Studien, die bei durchschnittlich älteren Kollektiven Harris-Scores von über 90% angeben (14, 21), liegt der mittlere Score in dieser Studie bei 87 ± 13 Punkten. Während die Patienten überwiegend zwischen 90 und 100 Punkten erreichen, liegen doch 12 Patienten bei einer Punktzahl von unter 80. Ein höherer Aktivitätsanspruch mag hier ebenso eine Rolle spielen, wie die innerhalb dieser arbeitsfähigen Patientengruppe immer wieder geäußerten Rentenbegehren. Den subjektiven Schmerzäußerungen steht der hohe Grad an Zufriedenheit bei 49 von 50 Patienten entgegen. Bei der qualitativen röntgenologischen Betrachtung zeigt sich unabhängig von der Gleitpaarung eine nur geringe Saumbildung um das Pfannenimplantat. Konventionell radiologisch waren weder eine Implantatmigration noch sonstige Lockerungszeichen zu verzeichnen.

Die Einbildröntgenanalyse EBRA stellt das einzige röntgenologische Messverfahren dar, das Implantatmigrationen mit einer Genauigkeit von 1 mm ohne Implantation metallischer Marker erfasst. Zur Durchführung der EBRA sind mindestens 4 Beckenübersichten erforderlich (10). Bei einer Nachuntersuchungszeit von 2 Jahren ist diese Voraussetzung gerade eben erfüllt. Andererseits hat die EBRA einen hohen prädiktiven Wert für spätere Implantatlockerungen (11). Mit der Einbildröntgenanalyse konnten je 2 Implantate aus beiden Gruppen nicht ausgewertet werden, was im üblichen Rahmen liegt. Von den verbleibenden 46 Implantaten zeigte sich bei einem Patienten mit einem PE-Inlay eine Implantatmigration von 1,7 mm nach kranial. In der Konsequenz wird der Patient weiter in jährlichem Abstand klinisch und radiologisch kontrolliert. Aussagekräftiger als die Anzahl der gewanderten Implantete ist die mittlere Implantatmigration des Gesamtkollektivs. Während sich bei der mediolateralen Migration kein signifikanter Unterschied zwischen den beiden Gruppen zeigt, ist die kraniale Migration der Keramik-Gruppe signifikant geringer. Obwohl es reizvoll wäre, zu spekulieren, dass das Keramik-Inlay auf Grund der breiteren peripheren Krafteinleitung in das knöcherne Becken eine geringere kraniale Migration bewirkt, sollte diese Schlussfolgerung auf Grund des kurzen Beobachtungszeitraumes und der Betrachtung von nur 25 % des Gesamtkollektivs zunächst unterbleiben. Insgesamt ist die Rate der Migration des PLASMACUPS gering (5).

Die dargestellten Ergebnisse stellen einen Zwischenstand dar. Den günstigen klinischen und radiologischen Resultaten steht ein revisionspflichtiger Randabbruch entgegen. Die längerfristigen Ergebnisse des gesamten Kollektivs bleiben abzuwarten. Die Versorgung von jungen aktiven Patienten mit großem Bewegungsumfang und -anspruch bleibt weiterhin ein Grenzbereich der aktuellen Implantatkonzepte. Insbesondere für Patienten mit sagittalem Bewegungsumfang von mehr als 120° können Empfehlungen zur Wahl des Implantats und zu seiner optimalen Positionierung nur eingeschränkt gegeben werden.

Literatur

1. Blömer W (1997) Design aspects of modular inlay fixation. pp. 95–104. In Puhl, W (ed.): Performance of the wear couple Biolox forte in hip arthroplasty. Enke, Stuttgart
2. Böhler M, Knahr K, Plenk H, Jr. et al (1994) Long-term results of uncemented alumina acetabular implants. J Bone Joint Surg Br 76: 53–59
3. Garcia-Cimbrelo E, Martinez-Sayanes JM, Minuesa A et al (1996) Mittelmeier ceramic-ceramic prosthesis after 10 years. J Arthroplasty 11: 773–781
4. Harris WH (1993) Keynote address: Clinical considerations. pp. 1–11. In Morrey BF (ed): Biological, material and mechanical considerations of joint replacement. Raven, New York
5. Hendrich C, Bahlmann J, Eulert J (1997) Migration of the uncemented Harris-Galante acetabular cup – results of the Einbildröntgenanalyse (EBRA) method. J Arthroplasty 12: 889–895
6. Hendrich C, Kaddick C, Pfaff HG, Willmann G (2000) Do Ceramic Liners Alter the Load Transmission of Modular Hip Sockets? pp. 54–60. In Willmann G, Zweymüller K (eds.): Proceedings of the 5th International Symposium Thieme, Stuttgart
7. Huo MH, Martin RP, Zatorski LE et al (1996) Total hip replacements using the ceramic Mittelmeier prosthesis. Clin Orthop 332: 143–150
8. Ilchmann T, Franzen H, Mjoberg B, Wingstrand H (1992) Measurement accuracy in acetabular cup migration. A comparison of four radiologic methods versus roentgen stereophotogrammetric analysis. J Arthroplasty 7: 121–127
9. Johnston RC, Fitzgerald RH, Harris WH et al (1990) Clinical and radiographic evaluation of total hip replacement. J Bone Joint Surg Am 72: 161–168
10. Krismer M, Bauer R, Tschupik J, Mayrhofer P (1995) EBRA: a method to measure migration of acetabular components. J Biomechanics 28: 1225
11. Krismer M, Stöckl B, Fischer M et al (1996) Early migration predicts late aseptic failure of hip sockets. J Bone Joint Surg Br 78: 422–426
12. Kwong LM, O'Connor DO, Sedlacek RC et al (1994) A quantitative in vitro assessment of fit and screw fixation on the stability of a cementless hemispherical acetabular component. J Arthroplasty 9: 163–170
13. Mahoney OM, Dimon JH (1990) Unsatisfactory results with a ceramic total hip prosthesis. J Bone Joint Surg Am 72: 663–671
14. Robinson RP, Deysine GR, Green TM (1996) Uncemented total hip replacement arthroplasty using the CLS stem: a titanium alloy implant with co-

rundum blast finish. Results of a mean 6 years in a prospective study. J Arthroplasty 11: 286–292
15 Russe W (1988) pp. 1–80 Röntgenphotogrammetrie der künstlichen Hüftgelenkspfanne. Huber, Bern
16 Schmalzried TP, Kwong LM, Jasty M et al (1992) The mechanism of loosening of cemented acetabular components in total hip arthroplasty. Analysis of specimens retrieved at autopsy. Clin Orthop 274: 60–78
17 Smith SE, Harris WH (1997): Total hip arthroplasty performed with insertion of the femoral component with cement and the acetabular component without cement. J Bone Joint Surg Am 79: 1827–1833
18 Widmer KH, Zurfluh B, Morscher EW (1997) Contact surface and pressure load at implant-bone interface in press-fit cups compared to natural hip joints. Orthopäde 26: 181–189
19 Willmann G (1998) Ceramics for total hip replacement – what a surgeon should know. Orthopaedics 21: 173–177
20 Winter M, Griss P, Scheller G et al (1992) Ten- to 14-year results of a ceramic hip prosthesis. Clin Orthop 282: 73–80
21 Zenz P, Pospisil C, Fertschak W. Schwägerl W (1995) 10 Jahre zementfreie Implantation von Hüfttotalendoprothesen unter Verwendung des Zweymüller-Schaftes. Z Orthop 133: 558–561

1.8 MPF Modular Press Fit Cup – The Concept, Experience and First Results

G. Scheller, A. Claus, B. Günther, H. Schroeder-Boersch, L. Jani

The Concept

When developing the cementless MPF-cup, the authors had set the following criteria as their aim: The cup should have a hemispherical shape, the inlays should be modular. There should be a high initial stability, the surface of the implant should provide a high amount of osseointegration to provide a secondary stability of the implant. The use of additional fixation elements and the use of a ceramic-ceramic bearing without polyethylen should be possible (Fig. **1**).

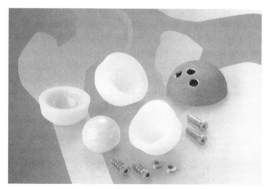

Fig. 1 MPF Modular Press Fit Cup.

The hemispherical shape of the cup allows a minimal bone resection because the geometry respects the normal anatomy of the acetabulum.

A modular inlay allows the surgeon to choose among different materials. If necessary, it is possible to use a dysplasia-inlay, and in revision surgery one only has to change the inlay in case of an osseointegrated titanium cup.

The superior primary stability is achieved by a combination of different features. The combination of different radii with different centres, and the same diameter of the reamer as that of the outer radius of the implant provides a form-fit and a press-fit over a large area. The oversize increases with the diameter of the cup and, thus, creates an equally strong press-fit starting with the smallest size and extending to the maximum size. The contact of the cup is reduced at the dome to provide a physiological distribution of forces. The sharp outer edge and the roughness of the surface of the cup also increases the primary stability. Biomechanical tests in a foam block model (3) substantiate the outstanding stability values of this hemispherical cemnetless cup (Fig. **2**). The lever-out force for the MPF-cup with 2 mm press-fit was measured with 29.35 Nm.

It should be possible to use additional fixation devices to increase primary stability, for example in revision cases or in patients with hip-dysplasia. Available are cancellouse screws and bolts having a rough surface, which are firmly connected to the titanium cup. Penetration of polyethylen particles can be avoided by closing the screwholes with titanium plugs.

The porous coating of the pure titanium grade 4 shell is produced using a vacuum plasma spray technology of pure titanium powder. The coating thickness is 400 um, the pore size distribution ranges between 40 um and 300 um, the open porosity varies between 20% and 40%. Fig. **3** shows the osseointegration of this surface in a minipig model after 12 weeks.

An important aim in the development of the MPF-Cup was the use of the ceramic-ceramic bearing without an intervening layer of polyethylen. Any additional material and any additional interface carries a certain risk of dislocation, movement, wear and fretting. The upper edge of the ceramic inlay should be completely supported by the metal shell to avoid any weak point and any impingement on the neck of the stem (Fig. **4 a, b**).

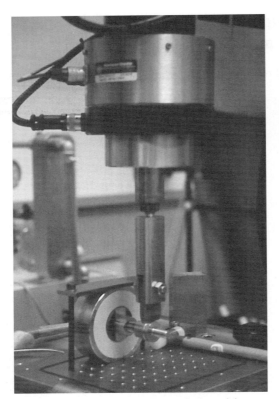

Fig. 2 Lever-out Test in the Foam Block Model.

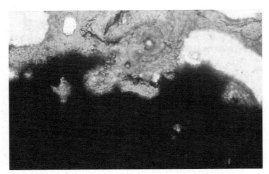

Fig. 3 Osseointegration of the Pure Titanium Plasmaspray in a Minipig Model after 12 Weeks.

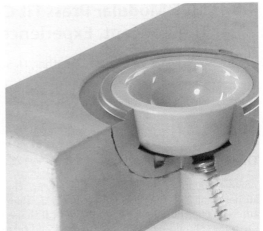

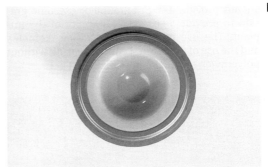

Fig. 4 a, b Ceramic Inlay with completely supported upper edge.

Table 1 Demographics

59 patients	
30 female	29 male
mean age	55.4
AVN	3
Dysplasia	7
Prim. Osteoarthritis	49

Material and Methods

Between November 1997 und January 1999, 59 primary total hip arthroplasties using the MPF-cup having a ceramic-ceramic bearing with a 28 mm diameter were performed in 59 patients. The study is conducted as a prospective series. Indication for the ceramic-on-ceramic hip replacement is that patients must be active and younger than 65 years. The ratio female/male was 30/29. The mean age was 55.4 years. The most common diagnoses were primary osteoarthriris, AVN was noted in 3 hips, secondary osteoarthritis with hip-dysplasia in seven cases (Table **1**).

The follow-up closed a year later, on January 31, 2000, and included 53 hips.

Results

Clinical results are evaluated using the Harris Hip Score (HHS) and the Score of Merle d'Aubigne.

The Harris Hip Score shows an improvement from 47.2 points preoperative to 96.0 points after one year. The Score of Merle d'Aubigne rose from 10.5 points to 17.1 points (Table **2**).

The radiographic evaluation showed no measurable migration or change in the inclination of a cup.

Radiolucent lines under 1 mm were observed in 6 patients in zone II, a complete remodelling of the initial gap at the dome of the cup was observed in 39 cases. All MPF-Cups were radiographically osseointegrated (Fig. **5a,b**).

At least as important as good short term results are the complications arising during this period. In our series we had one severe DVT and one secondary deep infection. As implant related complications we found 3 dislocations and one intraoperatively damaged ceramic inlay.

One dislocation occurred four weeks post-op following discharge from the hospital in a low seat with a flexion more than 110°. Following closed reduction, there were no further problem. The inclination of the cup measured was 43°. The second dislocation occurred in a case of hip-dysplasia 10 days postoperative during a external rotation and adduction movement. The patient suffered another dislocation after five weeks. Again following closed reduction, there were no further problems and the result after one year was very good. The inclination of this cup was 49°.

The third dislocation happened to a 50 years old woman with a body-weight of 117 kg and a

Table 2 Clinical Results

HHS preop 47.2	HSS 1 year 96.0
MDA preop 10.5	MDA 1 year 17.1

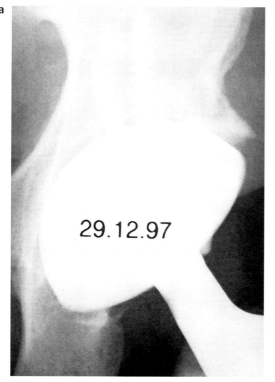 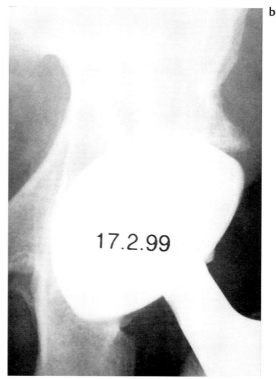

Fig. 5a,b Bone remodelling after one year.

Table 3 Complications

DVT	1
Secondary deep infection	1
Dislocations	3
Rim fracture CE-inlay	1

height of 1.68 m for the first time after 8 days. After an easy to perform closed reduction two reluxations occurred in the next 10 days under normal circumstances. Revision surgery was performed 21 days post-op, the ceramic-inlay was exchanged for a dysplasia inlay and a longer head was implanted. Subsequently, a deep infection occurred, which made a further revision surgery necessary. The inclination of this cup was also 49°.

In one of the first implantations a fracture of the rim of the ceramic inlay occured. The inlay was slightly tilted during the insertion into the cone of the metal shell (Fig. **6**). This type of complication is considered as a technical, operation-specific problem, and not as an implant failure. Since that time, we insert the ceramic inlay carefully by hand and fix it with a light tap of the hammer only after having carefully checked the position once more.

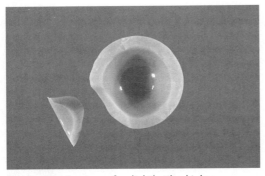

Fig. 6 Rim Fracture of a slightly tilted Inlay.

Discussion

The most important reason for using the ceramic-on-ceramic bearing in THA is to avoid the well-known problems of osteolysis around cup and stem, which is caused by polyethylen wear particles.

The low linear wear-rates of the alumina ceramic bearing under laboratory conditions is commonly accepted. Also former ceramic material of diverse quality with higher rates of wear showed no focal osteolysis after 25 years. Repeated luxations of ceramic hips may be critical. Therefore, an optimal cup position in relation to the stem is very important. By using a hemispherical cup the surgeon can change the position of the cup after the reaming process. A probe inlay gives the opportunity of checking reduction, testing stability and function before implanting the definitive inlay and head, or head and stem. The surgical technique for implanting the ceramic inlay may be critical, too. Further, a slightly tilted position of the ceramic inlay must be definitely avoided.

The migration of the Lindenhof or Mittelmeier cementless monobloc cups design is well known (2).

The ceramic surface of these implants was never osseointegrated. A recent publication (1) reported a higher rate of migration of cups with a ceramic inlay compared to identical cups with a PE-inlay. The measurements were carried out by means of EBRA I and a hemisherical cup with three pods. We see no rational reason for this behavior, but this reported phenomenon should be checked.

References

1 Boehler M, Mühlbauer M, Krismer M, Salzer M, Mayr G (1998) Migration Measurements of Cementless Acetabular Components: Value of Clinical and Radiographic Data. Orthopedics, 21(8), 897–900
2 Griss P, Claus A, Scheller G (1999) Analyse unserer Erfahrungen mit Keramik/Keramik-Hüftendoprothesen der ersten Generation (1974–1978) in Sedel L, Willmann G: Reliability and Long-term Results of Ceramics in Orthopaedics. Thieme, 43–47
3 Kuhn A, Scheller G, Schwarz M (1999) Primärstabilität zementfreier Press-fit-Hüftpfannen. In-vitro-Auskippversuche. Biomed. Technik, 356–359

1.9 2–4 Year Clinical Results with a Ceramic-on-Ceramic Articulation in a New Modular THR-System

G. A. Fuchs

Einleitung

Die Erfahrungen mit den Folgen von Abrieb-, Oxydations- und Lösungsvorgängen an Implantatoberflächen haben uns vor ca. 6 Jahren veranlasst, im Rahmen einer Neu-, bzw. Weiterentwicklung eines Hüftendoprothesensystems das Konzept der Modularität und damit die Auswahlmöglichkeit alternativer Biomaterialien mit einzubeziehen. Gleichzeitig konnte damit der aktuellen gesundheitspolitischen und wirtschaftlichen Entwicklung Rechnung getragen werden.

Bei der Suche nach alternativen Gleitmaterialien steht die Optimierung der tribologischen Eigenschaften konventioneller Gleitpaarung (z.B. Polyethylen/Metall) als wichtigste Voraussetzung im Vordergrund. Neben der Renaissance der Metallgleitpaarung (Metasul®) hat sich – durch ihre günstigen tribologischen und biologischen Eigenschaften – die Keramik-Gleitpaarung (Biolox forte®), abgesehen vom monolitischen System, klinisch bestens bewährt. Um aber den alternativen Einsatz von Hartpaarungen zu ermöglichen, musste eine neue Verankerungstechnik für die Pfannenschale entwickelt werden, die für das jeweilige Einsatzmaterial einen spezifischen Verklemmungsmechanismus besitzen muss. Unter Verwendung bewährter Implantatmaterialien für die Verankerungstechnik, wie Kobalt-Chrom-Molybdän- oder Titanlegierungen – je nach Implantationsart – konnte ein komplettes Hüftendoprothesensystem (BF) entwickelt werden, mit dem Vorteil gleichen Designs, identischen Op-Instrumentariums und daher breitem Indikationsspektrum, womit auch eine höhere Wirtschaftlichkeit in Bezug auf Lagerhaltung und Kosten erreicht werden konnte.

Berichtet wird nun über erste mittelfristige Ergebnisse von 1966 bis 1999 dieses neuen modularen Hüftendoprothesensystems (BF), mit Stahl- und Titanschäften einerseits und einer Titanpfannenschale andererseits. Die alternativen Inlay-Einsätze aus Polyethylen bzw. Aluminiumoxyd-Keramik können wiederum gegen Stahl- oder Aluminiumoxyd-Köpfe artikulieren. Das Op-Instrumentarium ist für alle Implantate gleich.

Material und Methode

Seit Fertigstellung und technischer Prüfung unseres Hüftendoprothesensystems (BF, Chiropro, Zirndorf) und vor allem der neuen Einsatztechnologie des Keramik-Inlays (CeramTec, Plochingen) wurden in der Zeit von 1996 bis 1999 in der Orthopädischen Klinik Bayreuth insgesamt 947 Hüftendoprothesen eingesetzt. Hiervon fanden 1996 noch teilweise andere Pfannentypen, z.B. vom Typ Sulmesh-Gitternetz (Griss) Verwendung, ansonsten wurden ausschließlich Implantate vom Typ BF-System verwandt. Der Anteil des neuen BF-HTEP-Systems an den insgesamt 947 implantierten betrug 921 BF-Schäfte bzw. 704 BF-Pfannen (Tab. 1 u. 2). Hierbei wurden 226 × die Keramik-Keramik-Gleitpaarung aus Biolox forte® verwendet. Das entspricht 32,1 % der BF-Gruppe bzw. 23,8 % von der gesamten Hüft-TEP-Summe (n = 947) (Abb. 1).

Die **Indikation** fand hierbei besonders für jüngere Patienten, in der Regel unter 65 Jahren mit längerer Lebenserwartung, Berücksichtigung. Das Durchschnittsalter lag bei der Keramik-Gleitpaarung bei 56,7 Jahren, gegenüber 67 Jahren der Gesamtgruppe. Die präoperative Diagnoseaufschlüsselung ist in Abb. 2 veranschaulicht.

Prothesenschaft

Die Form besteht bei der Zementversion in einem Geradschaft aus moderner S3O–Stahllegierung, mit relativ glattem Oberflächendesign, bei totaler Zementierung in Kombination mit einer sphäri-

1.9 Clinical Results with Ceramic-on-Ceramic Articulations in a Modular THR-System

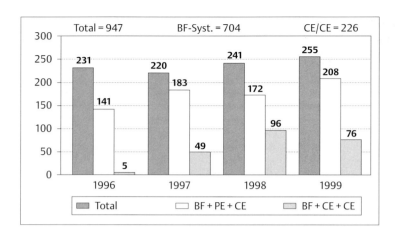

Abb. 1 Anteil der Keramik-Gleitpaarung seit 1996 an allen Hüft-TEPs (n = 947/24%) und an modularen BF-Hüft-TEPs (n = 704/32%). CE/CE-Gleitpaarung jeweils re. Säule.

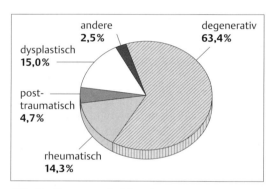

Abb. 2 Diagnoseaufschlüsselung

schen PE-Pfanne. Das Pendant für die zementfreie Verankerung ist eine gleichförmige Geradschaftprothese aus Titanlegierung mit säulenförmigem, erhabenem Oberflächendesign und einer Reintitan-Plasma-Spray-Beschichtung in der proximalen Verankerungszone von einer Porosität zwischen 200 und 400 µm. Die distale Schafthälfte ist poliert (Abb. 3). Der Konus-Halswinkel beträgt 140°, eine anfängliche Schenkelhalsantetorsion von 10° wurde zu Gunsten der Lagerhaltung und Wirtschaftlichkeit wieder verlassen. Neben Stahlköpfen können Aluminiumoxyd-Köpfe sowohl mit dem Durchmesser 28 wie auch 32 mm in 3 verschiedenen Halslängen benutzt werden.

Hüftpfanne

Die Pfanne besteht aus einer Titanlegierung ($TiAl_4V_6$) mit einer Rein-Titan-Oberfläche – wie der proximale Schaftanteil – mittels Plasma-

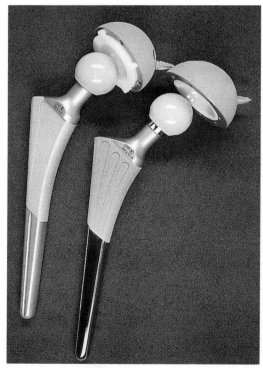

Abb. 3 BF-Hüft-TEP-System mit S30 Stahlschaft zur Zementierung (li.) und $TiAl_4V_6$-Schaft zur zementfreien Implantation (re.), proximal, wie bei der Pfannenrückseite, mit Rein-Titan im Plasma-Spray-Verfahren beschichtet.

Spray-Verfahren beschichtet (Abb. 4). In der Pfannendachzone ist im Winkel von 45° ein verschweißter selbstschneidender Zapfen zur Pri-

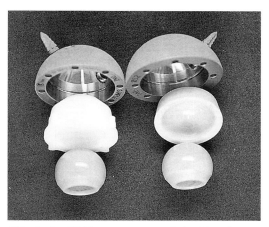

Abb. 4a, b BF-Pfanne zur zementfreien Verankerung und alternativer Einsatzmöglichkeit von Inserts aus
a Polyethylen – mit Schnappring- und Bohrlochverankerung
b Al_2O_3-Keramik – mit „umgekehrter", äquatornahen Konusklemmung

märstabilisierung angebracht. Weiterhin sind 3 multidirektionale Bohrungen zur fakultativen zusätzlichen Schraubenverankerung (siehe auch Revisions-Op) vorhanden. Das Pfannenzentrum besitzt eine Gewindebohrung, in die das Einschlaginstrument verankert wird.

Für die Verankerung des entsprechenden PE-Inlays ist einerseits eine Querrille in der mittleren Zirkumferenz der Pfanneninnenseite sowie auf der Außenseite, in der Eingangsebene, mehrere zirkulär angeordnete Bohrungen zur Aufnahme von Inlay-Zapfen zur zusätzlichen Rotationsstabilität vorgesehen. Für das Keramik-Inlay wurde wegen der vorgenannten Konstruktion eine „umgekehrte Konusklemmung" entwickelt, d.h. die Verklemmungszone liegt – entgegen anderer Systeme – äquatornah, wodurch mechanische Irritationen in der Pfannentiefe durch die o.g. Querrille vermieden werden können (Abb. **5**).

Der klinische und radiologische Verlauf wurde teils durch retrospektive Nachuntersuchungen und teils durch prospektive Verlaufskontrollen dokumentiert. Die retrospektiven Ergebnisse wurden im Zeitraum von 1994 bis 1998 kürzlich publiziert (3). Bei der prospektiven Verlaufsbeobachtung des BF-Hüft-TEP-Systems mit der Keramik-Gleitpaarung wurde wegen der speziellen Bedeutung der radiologischen und tribologischen Aspekte auf die klinischen Funktionsauswertungen weitgehend verzichtet.

Ergebnisse

A. BF-Hüft-TEP-System

Bei den 226 (24%) von insgesamt 947 in der Orthopädischen Klinik Bayreuth von 1996 bis 1999 implantierten Hüftendoprothesen mit Keramik-Gleitpaarung handelt es sich, neben 26 Schenkelhalsendoprothesen vom Typ DSP/ESKA-Cut (Abb. **6,7**), um ein neu entwickeltes BF-Hüft-TEP-System (Abb. **3**). Hiervon wurden 563 zementfrei eingesetzt, 254 teilzementiert (Hybrid) und 130 totalzementiert. Die 1 Jahr zuvor durchgeführten retrospektiven radiologischen und klinischen Nachuntersuchungen von 246 Hüften bei 230 Patienten mittels Auswertung mit dem Merle d'Aubigné-Score und eines eigens entwickelten Score of Daily Activity (SDA) ergaben ein Gesamtergebnis im 2–5-Jahreszeitraum von exzellenten und sehr guten Ergebnissen bei der zementfreien Version in 95%, bei der Hybrid-Anwendung in 93% und bei den totalzementierten Hüftendoprothesen in 89%.

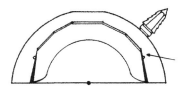 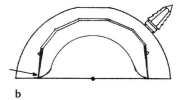

a b

Abb. 5a, b Schematische Darstellung der Al_2O_3-Insert-Verklemmung:
a in konventioneller Weise: dome-nahe Konusklemmung,
b im BF-System „umgekehrt", d.h. äquatornah, zur Vermeidung mechanischer Irritationen im dome-nahen Verklemmungsbereich (Bruchgefahr).

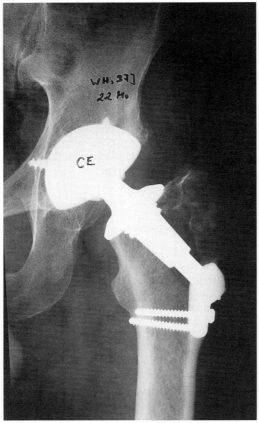
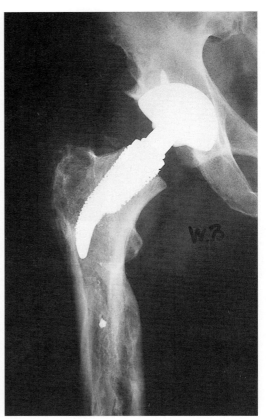

Abb. 6 2-Jahresergebnis nach Implantation einer Druckscheibenprothese bei einem 35-jährigen Rheumatiker, in Kombination mit der modularen BF-Pfanne und Keramikgleitpaarung.

Abb. 7 Versorgung einer posttraumatischen Coxarthrose mittels zementfreier SH-Prothese (ESKA-CUT®) in Kombination mit dem modularen BF-Pfannensystem mit Keramik-Gleitpaarung bei einem 39-jährigen Patienten nach beidseitiger Oberschenkeltrümmerfraktur und posttraumatischer/postoperativer Ostitis.

Komplikationen

Sichere Lockerungszeichen, Osteolysen, Schaftsinterungen etc. konnten in allen 3 Gruppen nicht festgestellt werden. Neben geringgradigen Pfannenmigrationen (unter 1 mm in 10 Fällen eines anderen Pfannentyps) fanden sich als spezifische Komplikationen 2 postoperative Luxationen in der zementfreien Gruppe und 3 Luxationen in der zementierten Gruppe. Tiefe Infekte traten in keinem Fall auf, insgesamt waren 7 oberflächliche Wundheilungsstörungen ohne weitere Konsequenzen aufgetreten. In diesem Krankengut (n = 230 Patienten) war die Keramik-Gleitpaarung noch unwesentlich vertreten (n = 5) und bei der Analyse – außer einer post-operativen Luxation – unauffällig.

Die in Tabelle **3** aufgeführten 3-maligen Revisionen wegen rezidivierenden postoperativen Luxationen (2 × PE, 1 × Keramik) hatten in allen 3 Fällen als gemeinsame Ursache einen zu flachen vorderen Pfanneneingangswinkel, d.h. eine zu geringe vordere Öffnung. Hierdurch kam es bei entsprechender gesteigerter Hüftbeugung zu dorsalen Luxationen. In einem Fall wurde lediglich das Inlay von Keramik auf PE mit einem Antiluxationsoffset gewechselt. Im 2. Fall die ganze Pfanne insgesamt neu positioniert und im 3. Fall, bei einer 82-jährigen Patientin (2 Jahre postoperativ!), ein dorsaler Antiluxationsring aus PE angebracht. Alle 3 Revisionen verliefen komplikationslos.

B. Ergebnisse mit der Keramik-Gleitpaarung

Bei den seit 1996 begonnenen prospektiven Verlaufsbeobachtungen an zementfreien Hüftendoprothesen mit Aluminium-Oxyd-Gleitpaarung (n = 226) standen weniger die klinischen Funktionstests als vielmehr eventuelle Folgen tribologischer Eigenschaften, spezifischer Komplikationen und radiologischer Besonderheiten im Vordergrund. Eine klinische Score-Beurteilung wurde daher nicht durchgeführt. Die Gesamtergebnisse dieses Patientenkollektivs, mit ausschließlich zementfreien Hüftendoprothesen sind, sowohl von der subjektiven Aussage, wie auch von den objektiven radiologischen und funktionellen Untersuchungsbefunden her, mit Ausnahme eines Falles, ausgesprochen zufriedenstellend. Diese entsprechen der retrospektiv nachuntersuchten Patientengruppe (n = 246) mit 129 zementfrei implantierten BF-HTEPs, mit 95% exzellenten/guten Ergebnissen (3). Bei dem einzigen Fehlschlag handelt es sich um eine 47-jährige extrem übergewichtige Rheumapatientin, die mit einer Druckscheibenprothese und einer BF-Pfanne mit CE-Gleitpaarung versorgt wurde. Postoperativ wurde hausärztlicherseits wegen eines akuten Rheumaschubes eine hochdosierte Cortisontherapie durchgeführt, mit der Folge der Implantatsinterung/-lockerung und einer notwendigen Revisionsoperation.

Komplikationen

Im übrigen Kollektiv traten im Beobachtungszeitraum von 4 Jahren (1996 bis 1999) bei den 92 männlichen und 134 weiblichen Patienten mit einem Durchschnittsalter von 56,7 Jahren (28 bis 71 Jahre), mit einem durchschnittlichen Follow-up von 20,7 Monaten, als Komplikationen 5 tiefe Beinvenenthrombosen, 2 oberflächliche Wundheilungsstörungen, 3 Trochanterfrakturen, 1 Schaftfraktur und 3 postoperative Luxationen (nach dorsal!) auf (Tab. **4**). Lockerungszeichen des Schaftes oder der Pfanne konnten, außer bei dem oben beschriebenen Fall, nicht nachgewiesen werden. Tiefe Infekte, Implantatbrüche, Migrationen und Resorptionszonen über 1 mm waren ebenfalls nicht nachweisbar. Eine Randabplatzung eines Keramik-Inlays konnte eindeutig durch Operateursbefragung und durch REM-Untersuchung der Bruchoberfläche als intraoperativer Handling-Fehler eingeordnet werden

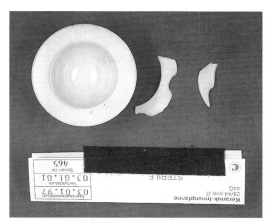

Abb. 8 Oberflächliche Kantenabscherung eines Keramik-Inserts durch unsachgemäße intraoperative Handhabung (Verkippung)

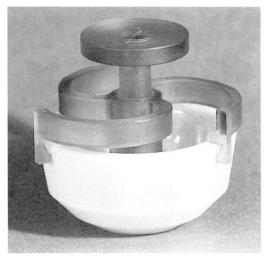

Abb. 9 Prototyp eines Kunststoff-Applikators zum sicheren Einsetzen des Inserts (Fa. CeramTec, Plochingen).

(Abb. **8**). Beim Einsetzen des Keramik-Inlays darf zur Vermeidung einer Schädigung auf keinen Fall eine Verkippung, geschweige ein weiterer Einschlagsversuch in dieser verkippten Stellung vorgenommen werden. Neuerdings wurde von CeramTec, ein Inlay-Applikator aus Kunststoff entwickelt, mit dessen Hilfe eine sorgfältige Insertion des Inlays vorgenommen werden kann (Abb. **9**).

Die bei entsprechend hohem Anteil an Dysplasiehüften (n = 15 %, Abb. 2) durchgeführten autologen Pfannenerkerplastiken zeigten radiologisch in allen Fällen ein unauffälliges Anwachsverhalten bei guter Abstützfunktion der Pfanne (Abb. 10). Die in den ersten Nachuntersuchungen (n = 246 HTEPs) noch in relativ hohem Anteil (27.9 %) nachweisbaren, klinisch allerdings unauffälligen kortikalen Hypertrophiezeichen an der Schaftspitze (stress-shielding), konnten seit der Polierung der distalen Schafthälfte bislang nicht mehr gesehen werden. Insbesondere traten keine periimplantäre Osteolysen als Zeichen einer „aggressiven Granulomatose" (2,4) als Ausdruck vermehrten Abriebs der Gleitpartner auf.

Diskussion

Die Kenntnisse der weitreichenden Folgen von Polyethylen- und PMMA-Abrieb einerseits und Oxydations-, Jonisations- und Lösungsvorgänge an Metalloberflächen andererseits (1,5,6,11) haben die Weiterentwicklung bzw. Suche nach alternativen Biomaterialien, speziell für hochbelastete Artikulationszwecke, in den letzten Jahren mehr oder weniger forciert. Ein wesentlicher Fortschritt kommt auf Grund der günstigeren tribologischen Eigenschaften der sogenannten **Hartpaarung** zu, sei es der Metall-Metallpaarung (Metasul®, 9) oder der von uns bevorzugten Keramik-Keramik-Paarung (Biolox forte®). Dass die Abriebbedingungen, sowohl vom physikalischen wie auch vom biologischen Gesichtspunkt her wesentlich günstiger als bei der konventionellen Gleitpaarung PE/Metall bzw. PE/Keramik sind, ist mittlerweile unumstritten (7,8,9,12).

Allerdings – und das dürfte auch in Zukunft ein limitierender Faktor bei der Anwendung sogenannter Hartpaarungen sein – sind die Kosten wesentlich höher gegenüber konventionellen Gleitpaarungen. Die Wahl alternativer Gleitpaarung (Hartpaarung), wie z. B. in unserem Krankengut, wird also einem bestimmen Patientenanteil, in der Regel jüngeren und aktiveren, evtl. auch extrem übergewichtigen Patienten, mit einer sonst zu erwartenden höheren Verschleißrate, vorbehalten bleiben. In jedem Fall ist, bei etwa gleich hoher operativer Komplikationsrate wie bei vergleichbaren konventionellen Hüft-TEP-Operationen, durch die technologische Weiterentwicklung der Keramik selbst (Biolox → Biolox forte) mit verminderten Abriebquoten (z. B.

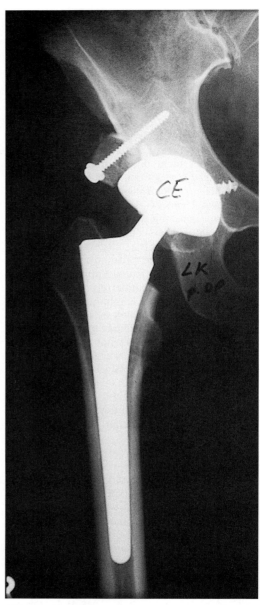

Abb. 10 Zementfreie Versorgung einer schweren Dysplasie-Coxarthrose mit dem modularen BF-System, Keramik-Gleitpaarung und autologer Pfannendachplastik bei einer 47-jährigen Patientin.

Biolox forte/Biolox forte < 0,001 mm gegenüber 0,1 mm/Jahr bei Biolox/Polyethylen) eine erheblich verbesserte Ausgangslage für die gewünschte Langzeitstabilität von Hüftendoprothesen geschaffen worden. Unterstützt wird diese durch die nachweislich bioinerte Materialeigenschaft der Aluminiumoxydkeramik, wie auch deren geringeren Partikelgröße mit entsprechend günstigeren morphologischen Gewebereaktion.

Ziel unserer vorliegenden Arbeit war es, in einem mittelfristigen Beobachtungszeitraum von bis zu 4 Jahren evtl. Vor- und Nachteile bei einem neuen, mit einer Keramikgleitpaarung kombinierten modularen Hüft-TEP-System (BF) durch prospektive Beobachtung zu analysieren.

Als Vergleich dient ein weiteres Patientenkollektiv (n = 230), das zuvor unter weitgehend identischen technologischen, biologischen und operationstechnischen Bedingungen retrospektiv klinisch und radiologisch nachuntersucht wurde und dessen Ergebnisse zwischenzeitlich publiziert worden sind (3). Der Anteil der Keramik-Gleitpaarung war hier allerdings für eine Aussage noch zu gering. Die Ergebnisse waren unter Auswertung mit dem Merle d'Aubigné-Score und einem eigens entwickelten SDA-Score (Score of Daily Activity) mit 89% in der vollzementierten, in 93% in der Hybridgruppe und mit 95% in der zementfreien Gruppe, im Mittel also in 92,3%, als exzellent und gut zu bewerten.

Vergleichend dazu sind die bis zu 4-jährigen prospektiven Beobachtungen an 226 zementfrei implantierten HTEPs mit Keramik-Gleitpaarung hinsichtlich klinischem Ergebnis, radiologischer Auswertung und spezifischer Komplikationsrate mit über 95% exzellenter und guter Ergebnisse eher noch überlegen, handelt es sich doch um ein selektioniertes, jüngeres Patientenkollektiv.

Als **Resumée** kann, auf Grund unserer bislang 14-jährigen Erfahrungen mit Keramik-Hüftköpfen einerseits und bis zu 4 Jahren mit der Keramik-Gleitpaarung andererseits, ein erheblicher Rückgang der Abriebproblematik und der damit verbundenen Komplikationen nach HTEP-Operationen verzeichnet werden. Somit besteht die begründete Erwartung bester Langzeitergebnisse, die allerdings zunächst abgewartet werden müssen.

Literatur

1 Davidson J A (1993) Characteristics of metal and ceramic total hip bearing surfaces and their effect on long-term ultra high molecular weight polyethylene wear. Clin. Orthop. Rel. Res. 294: 361–378
2 Fuchs G A (1995) Femurschaftosteolysen als begrenzender Faktor zementfreier Hüftendoprothetik? In: M Schmidt (Hrsg.) Die Metallpaarung „Metasul" in der Hüftendoprothetik. Hans Huber-Verlag, Bern 53–64
3 Fuchs G A, X Ren, J Wacker (1999) First 2–5 years results of single designed cemented and noncemented BF-prothesis in total hip arthroplasty. Orthop. J. China 6 (9): 711–715
4 Griss P, G A Fuchs, P Franke (1994) Die aggressive zystische Granulomatose des Femurschaftes – Polyaethylen-Krankheit als limitierender Faktor der Haltbarkeit zementfreier Hüftendoprothesenschäfte? Osteologie 3: 22–32
5 Schultz R, J H Johnson, R T Kiepura, D A Humphries (1987) Corrosion of titanium and titanium alloys. In: Metal Handbook: Corrosion, vol 13, Metals Park, American society for Metals, 669–706
6 Viegas M, L Abrantes, J Lecoer (1990) Metal materials biodegradation. A chronometric study. J. Mater. Sci. Mater. Med. 1: 105
7 Walter A (1992) On the material and tribology of alumina-alumina coupling for hip joint prosthesis. Clin. Orthop. Rel. Res. 282: 31–46
8 Walter A (1997) Investigation of wear couple Biolox forte/Biolox forte. In Puhl W (ed.) Performance of wear couple Biolox forte in hip arthroplasty. Enke-Verlag, Stuttgart
9 Weber B G (1992) Metall-Metall-Totalendoprothese des Hüftgelenkes – zurück in die Zukunft? Z Orthop. 130: 306–309
10 Willert H G, H Bertram, G H Buchhorn (1990) Osteolysis in alloarthroplasty of the hip – The role of UHMW polyethylene wear. Clin. Orthop. 258: 95–107
11 Willert H G, G H Buchhorn, M Semlitsch (1993) Particle disease due to wear of metal alloys – Findings from retrieval studies. pp 129–1, chapter 11. In: Biological, material and mechanical considerations of joint replacement: Current concepts and future direction. Morrey B (ed.) Raven Press, New York
12 Willmann G, H Kälberer, H G Pfaff (1996) Keramische Pfanneneinsätze für Hüftendoprothesen. Biomed. Technik 41, 4: 98–105

1.10 Peri-Acetabular Osteolysis in Press-Fit Ceramic-Ceramic and Ceramic-Polyethylene Total Hip Replacement: 5–7 Years Follow-Up

F. Bonicoli

Press-fit hip arthroplasties in the 1980s had excellent porous ingrowth (4,11), but about 5 years after implantation a high incidence of peri-prosthetic osteolysis is observed. This is due to the penetration into the bone-prosthesis interface of microdebris carried by synovial fluid (1,7,8,10, 11,12,18).

Compared to the acetabular cement-bone interface, porous ingrowth opposes a stronger barrier to the entrance into the metal-bone interface of synovial fluid and debris. However, synovial fluid and debris can follow other routes, eg rarified pelvic spongiosa, exposed areas of milled acetabulum and pre-existing osteo-arthritic cysts (geods) (12).

Even when debris-free, synovial fluid can cause osteolysis because of fluid hypertension (12,13) and, it seems, owing to the inflammatory mediators contained in it (9). Geods and rapidly destructive hip arthropathy could be so explained (9). Osteolytic potential is strongly enhanced when synovial fluid contains considerable quantities of micro-debris (18).

As of the beginning of the 1990s, press-fit prostheses were modified in order to minimise debris formation and their deleterious effects. These new-generation press-fit prostheses have more stable modular connections and their tribology is improved. Modern ceramic-ceramic coupling in these newer press-fit prostheses is the most wear-resistant. With these materials the wear rates are as low as 1 micrometer per year (2,14,16,17,19,21).

Ceramic-polyethylene couplings should also offer a high degree of resistance to wear thanks to the insert's thickness (over 6 mm) and to improved manufacturing, sterilisation and storage.

It will be interesting to see to what extent debris osteolysis occurs in new press-fit prostheses with a polyethylene insert.

Although it is too early to give a clear-cut answer to this question – because the time lapse since these devices were first implanted is too short – we believe this problem deserves to be addressed even with the data presently available.

We report radiological, surgical and histopathological assays of wear lesions in two types of new generation press-fit hip prostheses. One with ceramic-ceramic couplings, the other with ceramic-polyethylene couplings. All devices had been correctly implanted an average of 6 years previously.

Materials and Methods

During 1994 and 1995 in the Orthopaedics and Traumatology Unit of Lucca's Ospedale Civile (Italy), new generation press-fit total hip arthroplasties were performed in 120 patients. We re-evaluated 42 of these patients (28 women, 14 men, mean age 63 years, range 45–75 years), 21 patients had ceramic-ceramic couplings (Samo-Ceram-tec, see Fig. 1) and 21 had ceramic-polyethylene couplings. All patients received first implants, appropriately positioned (40–45° cup-inclination, 15–20° anteversion). All patients had primary or slight dysplastic osteoarthritis. All 42 patients had pelvis X-ray (centered on the symphysis pubica) and comparative CT of the acetabular roof. Component stability, radiolucent lines and zones of osteolysis were evaluated on the pelvis X-rays. Müller's template was used to measure the insert's linear wear (Fig. 2).

Spiral CT was used. Thin, 1–3 mm layers were examined in order to minimise artefacts due to radiological dispersion and in order to permit unequivocal interpretation of the images.

On CT, osteolysis was ascribed to wear debris only if images of osteolysis were neither surrounded by sclerosis, nor were present before surgery.

In the two patients who required surgical re-intervention (see below), the degree of the com-

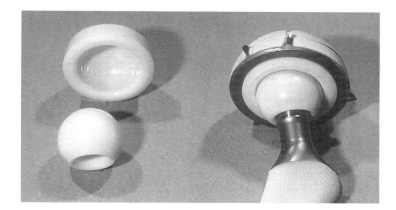

Fig. 1 Cementless socket and stem made of titanium covered with HA manifactured by SAMO – Cadriano Emilia (Italy). Ceramic BIOLOX FORTE insert and 28 mm head manifactured by CeramTec Plochingen (Germany).

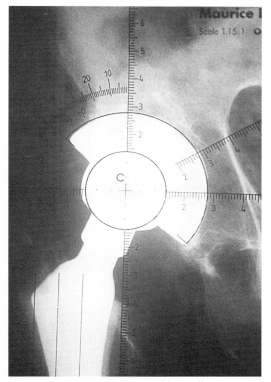

Fig. 2 Linear wear is measured by Muller Hip Template.

ponents' osteointegration, the state of the modular connections, the thickness and the appearance of the head's and the insert's weight-bearing surfaces were directly evaluated. In addition, histology of immediately peri-prosthetic soft-tissues was obtained.

Results

42 cases, mean follow-up 60 months (range 48 – 72 months).

A Ceramic-ceramic group (21 cases)

I Radiological findings (21 cases)

1. X-rays of the pelvis and of the arthroplasty did not show in any case excentricity of the head, nor debris osteolysis.
2. In one case a large geod present before surgery remained unchanged (Figs. **3** and **4**).
3. In no case was radiolucency detected.

II CT (21 cases)

Comparing CT images of the roof of the acetabulum on the operated side with that on the other side gave the following results:
1. Normal bone architecture in 20 cases.
2. Unchanged geod with respect to preoperative appearance 1 case.
3. Osteolysis: no case.
4. Extra-osseus cysts: no case.

III Surgical findings (1 case)

Female patient, 57 years of age, underwent total hip replacement 5 years previously, recently re-operated to remove peri-prosthetic ossifications which hampered flexion beyond 70° (Fig. **4**). Preoperative X-rays and CT imaging showed a large geod in the acetabular roof. 5 years postoperative X-ray (Fig. **5**) and CT images showed the geod's unchanged aspect. Intraoperative the cup and

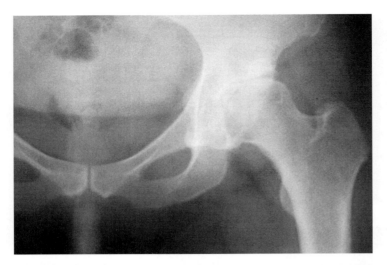

Fig. 3 Active female, 57. Osteoarthritis of the left hip with big sovra-acetabular geod.

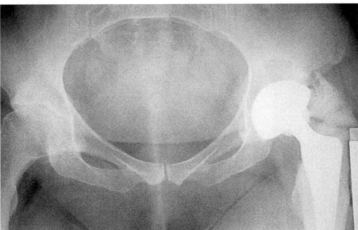

Fig. 4 Same patient of Fig. **3**, after 64 weeks from new generation ceramic-ceramic press-fit total hip replacement. The sovra-acetabular geod is not changed. A big ossification, restricting the hip ROM over 70 degrees of flexion, is present.

the shaft were stable, ceramic components were in excellent conditions, peri-prosthetic soft-tissues appeared to be normal. Histology did not detect any debris or giant poly-nucleated cells, but histiocytes were present (Fig. **5**).

B Ceramic-polyethylene group (21 cases)

I Radiological results (21 cases)

Results of pelvis X-ray and arthroplasty X-ray:
1. Centred head in 20 cases, excentric (1 mm) head in 1 case, Fig. **6**).
2. No peri-acetabular osteolysis.
3. No case of radiolucency.

II CT findings (21 cases)

Normal bony architecture in 20 cases.
No case of extra-osseus cysts.

III Surgical findings (1 case)

Female patient, 70 years of age, 5 years after implantation of a total ceramic-polyethylene arthroplasty because of right-sided degenerative joint disease. Repeated surgery after recurrent luxation (twice). The first luxation occurred six weeks after surgery, the second episode five years later after a fall (Fig. **7**). The polyethylene insert and the ceramic head were retrieved. Fragments of the pseudo-capsule were subjected to

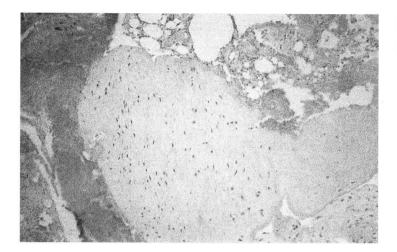

Fig. 5 Same patient of Fig. 4. Histology: debris and polinuclear giant cells are absent. Many histiocytes are visible.

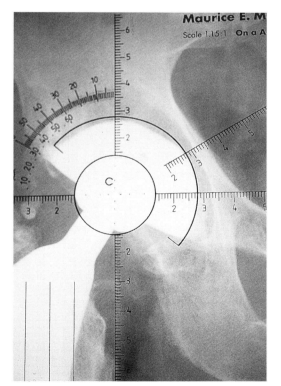

Fig. 6 Active male, 59. After 60 weeks from new generation ceramic-polyethylene press-fit total hip replacement: 1 mm of wear (linear wear 0.2 mm/yr).

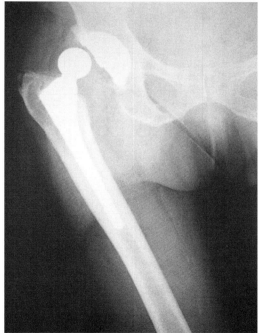

Fig. 7 Active female, 70. Recurrent (twice) dislocation of new generation ceramic-polyethylene press-fit total hip replacement, implanted 61 weeks before.

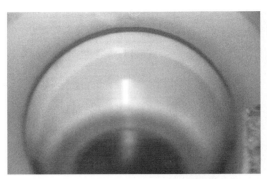

Fig. 8 Same patient of Fig. 7. Polar ovalization of polyethylene insert: transverse diameter 28 mm, vertical diameter 28,7 mm (linear wear: 0.14 mm/yr).

histologic examination. The ceramic head was undamaged, while the inside of the insert was slightly ovalised, its transverse diameter measured 28 mm and its longitudinal diameter 28.7 mm, (wear rate 0.14 mm/year) (Fig. **8**). Histology revealed plenty of fragments of bi-refrangent substance measuring 0.5–5 micrometer identical to bits of polyethylene, many histiocytes and giant polynucleate cells (Fig. **9**). In this patient periprosthetic bone of the acetabular roof appeared normal on pelvis X-ray and CT.

Discussion

Wear of the ceramic components is often due to the vertical cup's inclination or to poor quality ceramic or to taper mismatch (6). But these problems are now overcome by improvements along the surgeon's learning curve and by top quality modern materials (14, 16, 17, 19, 20, 21).

Since the clinical course of debris peri-prosthetic osteolysis remains silent for years, methods capable of detecting pre-clinical damage are useful. Peri-prosthetic osteolysis appears as round radiotransparent images without peri-focal sclerosis on conventional X-rays and CT.

Perhaps CT findings are positive earlier than conventional X-ray examinations, because of CT's higher sensitivity, although this point is still unproven. CT has not yet been widely adopted because interpretation of images distorted by metal's radiographic dispersions is difficult. CT images of the acetabular roofs are however easily interpreted and are hence useful to establish if and when revision surgery is indicated and to guide in the choice of the best surgical strategy.

An X-ray study of acetabular roofs 6 years after implantation of old generation press-fit arthroplasties with metal-polyethylene coupling, osteolysis was found in 20% of the cases (8). Osteolytic areas always lacked perifocal sclerosis.

CT images of debris osteolysis appear as "beehive" (Fig. **10**) and "oil stain" patterns (Fig. **11**). In some cases CT showed extra-osseous cysts (Fig. **12**), which at surgery were filled by pitch-black synovial fluid, confirming Schmalzried's observation that the boundaries of the artificial joint include the entire prosthesis even in well-fixed components (12).

Debris osteolysis can be mistaken for osteoarthritic geods. The latter are due to the penetration of high pressure synovial fluid into sub-

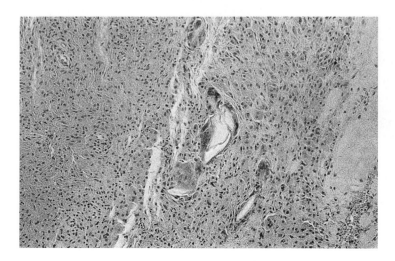

Fig. 9 Same patient of Fig. 7. Histology: many fragments of bi-refrangent material (0.5–5 micron in size) and polynuclear giant-cells are present.

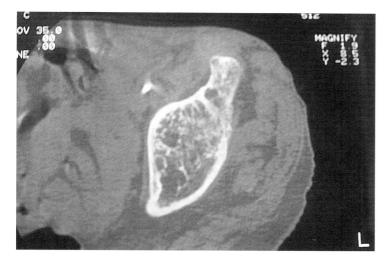

Fig. 10 Acetabular roof CT of old generation metal –polyethylene press-fit total hip replacement, implanted 67 weeks before. Honeycomb-like osteolysis.

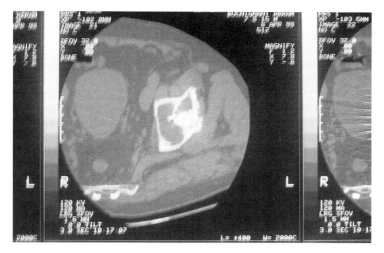

Fig. 11 Acetabular roof CT of old generation ceramic – polyethylene press-fit total hip replacement, implanted 70 weeks before. Oilstain-like osteolysis.

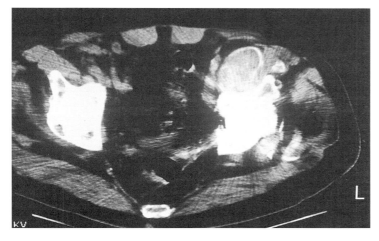

Fig. 12 Acetabular roof CT of left-side old generation metal (cr-co) – polyethylene press-fit total hip replacement, implanted 72 weeks before. Bulky endopelvic extra-osseous cyst containing black synovial fluid.

chondral bone through cartilage micro-cracks. They appear as inflated-balloon-like hypertransparent areas, usually bordered by sclerosis (3, 13). However if the synovial fluid contains debris, macrophage activation and osteoclast-stimulated bone resorption reduce perifocal sclerosis (5, 10,11). Comparison with pre-operative X-rays helps in differential diagnosis (Figs. **3** and **4**).

Geods must be considered areas at risk of debris accumulation and can collapse.

Osteolysis and destructive processes are absent in new generation press-fit ceramic-ceramic arthroplasties because debris production is insignificant. Therefore geods and small areas of missing bone-prothesis contact are less dangerous.

New-generation press-fit ceramic-polyethylene arthroplasties are more wear-resistant than older ones.

Obvious signs of peri-prothesic osteolysis were so far not detected by means of conventional X-rays and CT. However, polyethylene wear may still occur, as substantiated by the case in our series in which the head was excentric (Fig. **6**). Moreover, surgical findings in two of our cases confirm that debris, absent in ceramic-ceramic prostheses, are present in ceramic-polyethylene ones.

Conclusions

It is unclear whether acetabular roof CT can detect periprosthetic osteolysis earlier than conventional X-rays can, but it is certain that CT is more accurate in the exact planning of revision surgery. In addition, CT allows the surgeon to directly monitor over the years the quality of implanted prosthetic materials and hence timely draw appropriate consequences.

Press-fit ceramic-ceramic arthroplasties 6 years post-implantation did not show any signs of osteolysis, there was no evidence of wear and osteointegration was preserved. Nowadays a ceramic-ceramic coupling seems to be the best means to withstand wear.

The results of new generation press-fit ceramic-polyethylene arthroplasties are improved compared to older ones. Indeed six years post-implantation, osteo-integration is excellent and there is no evidence of peri-prosthetic osteolysis. However, since some material wear on these prostheses still occurs, further close observation has to be continued in the future.

References

1. Agins HJ, Alcock NW, Bansal M et al (1988): Metallic Wear in failed titanium-alloy total hip replacements: a histological and quantitative analysis. J Bone Joint Surg Am 70: 347–353
2. Boehler M, Knahr K. Salzer M et al (1994): Long term results of uncemented alumina acetabular implants. J Bone Joint Surg Br 76, 53–59
3. Carreri G, Urso S, Barbabella R et al (1996): Osteofitosi periarticolare e lesioni cistico-geodiche nella coxartrosi. Diagnostica per immagini. Ital J Orthop Traum Suppl. I: 197–204
4. Di Maio F, Lewallen DG, McGann WA et al (1996): Hip and Pelvis Reconstruction. Orthopaedic Knowledge Update 5: 389–426
5. Goldring SR, Schiller AL, Roelke K et al (1986): The synovial-like membrane at the bone-cement interface in loose total hip replacements and its proposed role in bone lysis. J Bone Joint Surg Am 65: 575–584
6. Gossens M (1999): The Transcend Alumina Ceramic Hip Articulation System. In: Sedel L, Willmann G (ed). Reliability and Long-term Results of Ceramics in Orthopaedics. 4th International CeramTec Symposium. Thieme, Stuttgart
7. Harris WH, Schillen AL, Schollen J-M et al (1976): Extensive localized bone resorption in the femur following total hip replacement. J Bone Joint Surg Am 58: 612–618
8. Kim YH, Kim VEM (1993): Uncemented porous-coated anatomic Hip Replacement: Results at six years in a consecutive series. J Bone Joint Surg Am 75: 6–13
9. Komiya S, Inoue A, Sasaguri Y et al (1992): Rapidly destructive Arthropathy of the Hip. Studies on Bone and Resorptive Factors in Joint Fluid with a Theory of Pathogenesis. Clin Orthop 248: 273–282
10. Maloney WJ, Peters P, Engh CA et al (1993): Severe Osteolysis of the Pelvis in Association with Acetabular Replacement without Cement. J Bone Joint Surg Am 75: 1627–1635
11. Rubash HE, Sinha RK, Shanbhag AS et al (1998): Pathogenesis of Bone Loss after Total Hip Arthroplasty. Clin Orthop North America 29: 173–186
12. Schmalzried TP, Jasty M, Harris WH (1992): Periprostetic Bone Loss in total Hip Arthroplasty. J Bone Joint Surg Am 74: 849–863
13. Schmalzried TP, Guttmann D, Grecula M et al (1994): The Relationship between the Design Position an Articular Wear of Acetabular Components Inserted without Cement and the Development of Pelvic Osteolysis. J Bone Joint Surg Am 76: 677–688

14 Sedel L (1999): Evolution of Alumina/Alumina implants. In: Sedel L, Willmann G (ed) Reliability and Long-term Results of Ceramics in Orthopaedics. 4th International Ceram Tec Symposium Thieme, Stuttgart 2–6
15 Taylor SK, Serekian P, Manley M (1998) Wear Performance of a Contemporary Alumina – Alumina Bearing Couple Under Hip Joint Simulation, 44th Ann. Meeting, Orthop Res Soc, March 15–19, 1998, New Orleans, Louisiana 51–59
16 Toni A, Terzi S, Sudanese A et al (1995): The use of Ceramic in Prosthetic Hip Surgery. The State of the Art. Chir Org Mov 80: 125–137
17 Walter A (1992): On the Material and the Tribology of Al/Al Coupling for Hip Joint Prostheses Clin Orthop Rel Res 282: 31–46
18 Willert HG, Semlitsch M (1977): Reactions of the articular capsule to wear products of artificial joint prostheses. J Biomed Mater Res 11: 157–164
19 Willmann G (1998): Ceramics for Total Hip Replacements – What a Surgeon should know. Orthopedics 21: 897–900
20 Willmann G, von Chamier W (1998): The Improvements of the Materials Properties of BIOLOX Offer Benefits for THR. Bioceramics 11: 649–652
21 Willmann G (1999): Ceramic Ball Head Retrieval Data. In: Sedel L, Willmann G (ed). Reliability and Long-Term Results of Ceramics in Orthopaedics. 4th International CeramTec Symposium. Thieme, Stuttgart, 62–63

1.11 Do Ceramic Liners Alter the Load Transmission of Modular Hip Sockets?

C. Hendrich, C. Kaddick, H. G. Pfaff, G. Willmann

Abstract

New modular hip sockets allow the use of inlays from different materials e.g. polyethylene, ceramic or sandwich-type. By the use of a ceramic insert instead of conventional polyethylene the stiffness of the complete acetabular implant is enhanced. This study describes the effect of a ceramic inlay upon the load transfer into the bony acetabulum using a Finite Element-analysis.

In a polyethylene inlay the strain energy density is concentrated at the dome of the cup, for sandwich-type and even more for ceramic liners a broader strain distribution into the periphery of the cup can be observed.

The clinical relevance of this results cannot be estimated yet. However a broader strain distribution may allow a more natural way of load transmission via the flanges of the implant.

Introduction

In the case of modern total hip replacement a tendency towards using hemispherical titanium-alloy shells with polyethylene liners can be observed which have shown superior mid- and longterm results [1]. In contrast threaded acetabular cups demonstrate worse clinical results and a higher rate of implant migration [2,3]. In spite of this progress, because of the risen life expectancy, the limited durability of the acetabular component remains the main problem on the field of total hip replacement [4]. Osteolysis induced by wear particles is considered to be the decisive cause for acetabular component loosening [5]. In order to avoid polyethylene wear ceramic-ceramic bearing surfaces have been used in Europe for almost two decades which, in comparison to conventional bearing surfaces, show a by several dimensions lesser wear [6,7]. The first generations of these acetabular components were without exception monolithic [8,12], for which the longterm results were mostly rather disillusioning [13,16]. Based on the explanted components the superior attributes concerning the minimized wear of the ceramic bearing surfaces [13,17] and the complete absence of particle induced osteolysis [18] could indeed be documented but on the other hand in the case of the cementless ceramic monolithic implants multiple fibrous fixations with simultaneously enhanced implant migration rates were observed [11,19,20]. Several reasons are made responsible for the high rate of radiologically unstable and migrated implants. Besides the insufficient material quality of the early ceramic [11] especially the threaded acetabular designs are mentioned [15]. Other reasons concerning the failure that are being discussed are the lack of porosity of the implant surface in contact with bone and the, in comparison to the spongy bone, much higher stiffness of the monolithic ceramic acetabular components [16].

Modern acetabular cup designs are modular, consisting of a metal shell and a polyethylene liner. For the alternative use of ceramic inserts new kinds of fixation had to be designed. Using the experience with the Morse taper fixation for ceramic ball heads an appropriate taper fixation also for the liner was designed which can be applied both in the case of ceramic and polyethylene inserts. For ceramic liners this type of fixation has proved to be reliable since 10 years [21]. This way the attractive tribological properties of the aluminum-on-aluminum coupling can be combined with the potential for good osseointegration of the metal-alloy cup [22].

However when using the ceramic inserts in metal shells the stiffness of the modular implant is enhanced in comparison to liners made of polyethylene [23]. The stiffness is correlated to the elastic modulus, the geometry, and wall thickness of the metal shell, which in current cup designs is very similar or even identical for both ceramic and polyethylene liners. While overall stiffness of a cup with a polyethylene insert is dominated by the metal shell because of its extremely high elastic modulus and the wall thickness of more than 4 mm the overall stiffness of a cup with a ceramic liner is dominated by the ceramic component [23].

The clinical significance of this enhanced stiffness cannot be calculated yet. While the shock absorption capacity of the actabular cup has only a minor effect compared to the elasticity of the whole extremity [23] the effect of the liner on the load transmission into the bony acetabulum is not known yet. To assess the strain distribution pattern in the present study a Finite Element- (FE-)analysis of three different acetabular liners (polyethylene, ceramic and sandwich-type of ceramic-in-polyethylene) within a titanium-alloy acetabular shell was performed.

Materials and Methods

Taper fixation of ceramic liners

Using the experience with the Morse taper fixation of ceramic ball heads also a taper fixation for the liners was developed in 1986. In the beginning the taper angle was 5°43′ (taper 1:10). In revision arthroplasty a ceramic liner fixed with this taper cannot be removed from the metal shell easily. Therefore four years ago the taper angle was changed (Fig. 1a). In all new concepts the angle is about 18° (taper 1:3) [21]. For revision purposes the insert can be removed by a hammer stroke on the rim of the metal shell. Details about the design of ceramic liners, combination with various metal shells, testing and reliability have been published recently [21,24]. An alternative to an all ceramic insert is a sandwich solution consisting of a ceramic liner molded into a polyethylene inlay (Fig. 1b). Clinical trials with this sandwich concept started about three years ago [25].

Finite Element-analysis

For the three-dimensional FE-analysis, two different types of mechanical boundary conditions were used: The simulation of a well ingrown cup was performed for three implant types as described in detail below. To gain information about the response to external deformations caused by

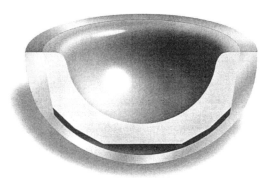

Fig. 1a Morse taper fixation of ceramic liners at a taper angle of about 18° (taper 1:3).

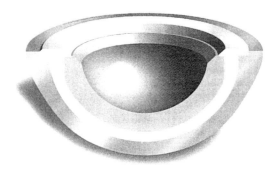

Fig. 1b Sandwich concept with a ceramic liner molded in polyethylene within the metal shell.

deformations of the acetabulum itself, a second FE-model was set up consisting of three implant types externally put under stress by a series of radial forces.

Strain energy density caused by the resulting hip force is calculated using a titanium-aluminum-vanadium metal shell for all implant types. Type 1 is defined by a polyethylene liner within a titanium-alloy metal back in clinical use now. Type 2 consists of a ceramic liner fixed by a Morse taper in a titanium-alloy metal shell of identical dimensions. Type 3 is a sandwich construction consisting of a ceramic liner molded into a polyethylene liner combined with a titanium-alloy metal shell (Fig. 2).

The metal cup is surrounded by a thin layer of subchondral bone (1 mm) followed by cancellous bone (5 mm) and a second layer of cortical bone (1 mm) (Fig. 3). The corresponding material characteristics are listed in Table 1.

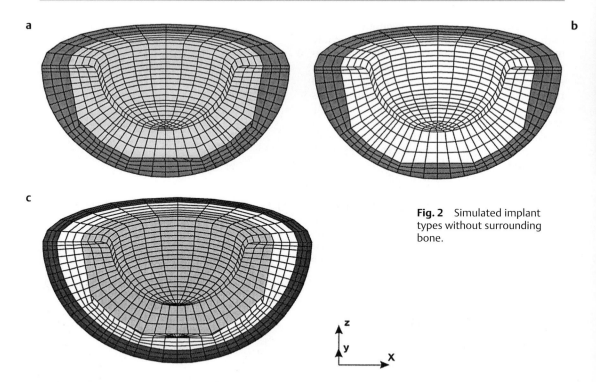

Fig. 2 Simulated implant types without surrounding bone.

Table 1 Material properties used for the FE-simulation

material	Young's modulus [Gpa]	Poisson ratio [-]
Ti6Al4 V	105	0.3
polyethylene	0.7	0.3
ceramics	380	0.23
subchondral bone	0.7	0.3
cancellous bone	0.5	0.2
cortical bone	6.2	0.33

The implants as well as the surrounding bone are modeled axisymmetrically. Hip load is applied axially (0°), in 20° inclination and in 40° inclination. To avoid localized stresses caused by unphysiologically applied forces, a ball was simulated and contact between the ball and the insert was enabled. The applied force was set at 3.0 kN. The cortical bone is fixed at the outer surface by boundary conditions.

Strain energy density was calculated according to

$$\text{SED} = \frac{1}{2}\bar{\varepsilon} \cdot \bar{\delta} \left[\frac{\text{N}}{\text{mm}^2}\right]$$

$\bar{\varepsilon}$: local strain tensor
$\bar{\delta}$: local stress tensor

To investigate the influence of external deflections representing the deformation of the acetabulum *in vivo*, a set of radial forces was applied to all implant types without simulating the surrounding bone (Fig. **4**). To avoid unrealistic defor-

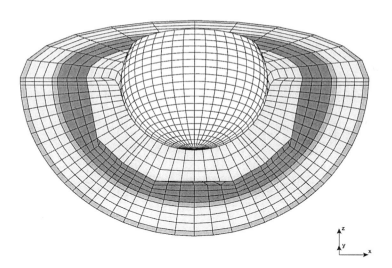

Fig. 3 Complete FE-mesh including surrounding bone and ball to apply external loads.

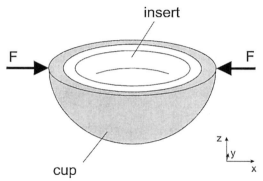

Fig. 4 FE-model to compare the structural stiffness of different implant types at radial loading conditions.

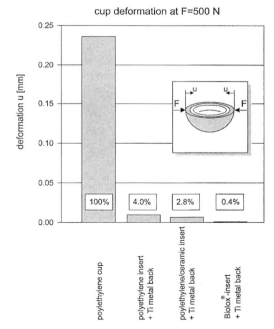

Fig. 5 Comparison of structural stiffness at radial loading conditions for different types of acetabular cups.

mations of the metal shell, the forces were applied using a set of n = 8 nodes on each side. The sum of forces was set to 500 N each. The resulting deflection at maximum load was assumed to represent the structural stiffness of the implant types investigated here.

Results

In order to compare the structural stiffness of the implants simulated a cup made of polyethylene without any metal backing was defined to be 100%. Relating to this, a metal shell leads to a reduction in terms of stiffness to 4%. A sandwich-type insert made of ceramic-in-polyethylene I was calculated to have 2.8% of the stiffness compared to the polyethylene cup without metal backing. Using a ceramic liner alters the stiffness to 0.4% (Fig. 5).

The external load applied by a ball has to be transmitted to the surrounding bone by the acetabular cup implant. Due to the different types of

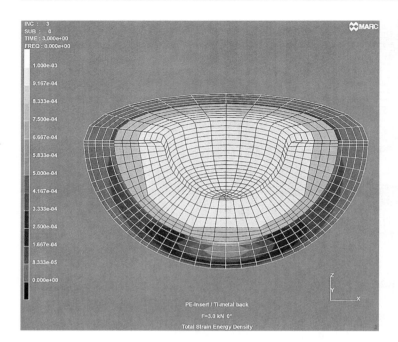

Fig. 6 Strain energy density for a polyethylene liner loaded axially at F = 3 kN.

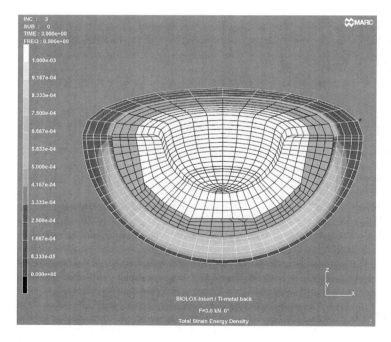

Fig. 7 Strain energy density for a ceramic liner loaded axially at F = 3 kN.

fixation of the insert, the pathway of the forces is altered. Regarding polyethylene liners in clinical use now, direct contact between the liner and the metal shell all over the backward side leads to a direct transmission of forces (Fig. 6). Due to this effect, the strain energy density is concen-

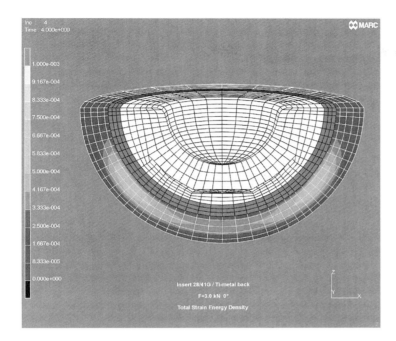

Fig. 8 Strain energy density for a sandwich-type liner made of ceramic-in-polyethylene loaded axially at F = 3 kN.

trated at the direction of the external load. The maximum strain energy density is calculated to be about 1.00 MPa.

Simulating a Morse taper fixation between the ceramic liner and the metal shell, the load has to be transferred more distally. The metal shell causes a broader distribution of pressure and, in consequence of strain energy density. It has to be noted that the difference in structural stiffness also plays an important role in the distribution of the different forms of stress (Fig. 7). The maximum strain energy density was found to be about 0.85 MPa.

The combination of both types of liners is realized by using a ceramic-in-polyethylene construction. The polyethylene acts as a dampening element between the ceramic articulation and the metal shell. In consequence the maximum strain energy density is located circularly at the mid part of the implant (Fig. 8). The maximum strain energy density is about 0.58 MPa.

Changing the inclination of the load leads to an asymmetrical shift of the stress distributions. The impact of load inclination on the shift corresponds to the type of fixation. Simulating polyethylene liners, the maximum remains at the proximal center region of the acetabulum (Fig. 9). In contrast, simulating a ceramic liner the distribution of the strain energy density becomes elliptically shaped and shifts distally (Fig. 10). The results for 20° inclination correspond to the changes in strain energy density described above. As expected, the local maximum was found between the maximum calculated for 0° inclination and 40° inclination.

Discussion

Clinical experience and histological investigations on retrieved ceramic heads and sockets prove that the rate of wear may be as low as 0.005 mm per year if neither the stem nor the cup has loosened [6,26]. For the ceramic-ceramic coupling the taper fixation of the insert proved to be very reliable. This concept has been used since 10 years (Fig. 1a). So far more than 2 million ceramic femoral heads and far more than 50,000 acetabular ceramic liners have been implanted [7]. Medium-term clinical and radiological results of the taper-fixed ceramic liners prove to be excellent [27,28].

The purpose of the present study was to investigate the influence of the type of liner within a metal-alloy cup on the stress distribution in the acetabular region. Due to the fact that upcoming

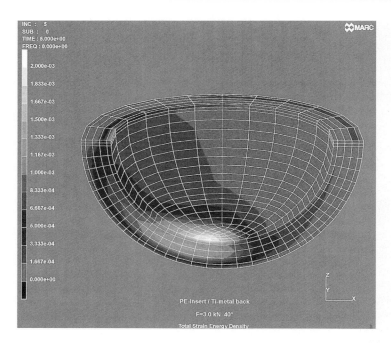

Fig. 9 Strain energy density for a polyethylene liner at a load of F = 3.0 kN inclined 40°.

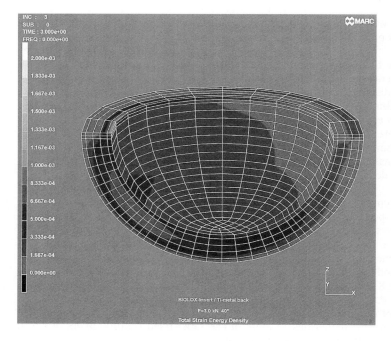

Fig. 10 Strain energy density for a ceramic liner at a load of F = 3.0 kN inclined 40°.

aluminum-on-aluminum bearings require new types of fixation, there is no data available comparing traditional types of fixation to the taper fixation of ceramic inserts available yet. In comparison to a polyethylene liner using a ceramic insert enhances the overall stiffness of the modular cup implant [23]. An alteration of stress distribution by the use of different liner materials can therefore be assumed.

In order to investigate the interaction between acetabular components and the underlying anatomic structures a number of different approaches can be made: first of all, an experimental setup using cadavers with simulated muscle action and external loads allows to simulate *in vivo* conditions. The results can be expressed in terms of deflection measured by linear transducers or strain measured by strain measurement gages or photoelasticity. The results are limited by the number of muscles and ligaments involved as well as by restrictions of the measurement techniques. Determination of strains is limited to the surface of the specimen.

The Finite Element-simulation is already well established in biomechanical research. Nevertheless there are also some limitations caused by the method itself: due to the increase in computing time the model refinement as well as the simulation of the contact conditions is limited. This fact can be taken into account by focusing the investigation on well defined, isolated problems. The decrease of impact concerning the whole anatomic structure leads to an increase in precision concerning the local mechanical interactions.

Finite Element-analysis of the pelvic bone has been performed by different authors [29–31]. Most of those studies are limited to mechanical effects caused by muscle activity and external loads while walking. The complexity of the model limits the results to a macroscopic point of view. More detailed investigation of the acetabular region has been performed by Dalstra 1993, Rapperport 1987, Weinans 1993 and Levenston 1993 [32–35].

In general, the acetabulum will be deformed in medial direction simulating *in vivo* conditions of single-leg stance, normal gait or stair climbing. It has been shown previously that a metal backing does not influence the resulting micromotions to the extent expected after theoretical investigations [30].

Contact pressures ranging from 8 MPa (normal gait) to 13 MPa (stair climbing) have been reported [29,30]. It has to be taken into consideration that the validity of the calculations is limited by the rough modeling of the FE-simulation. The contact pressure at the acetabular rim may be influenced due to this fact. Due to the bending of the acetabulum, pressure will dominate the outer surface of the implant. This fact enables the simplifications of two-dimensional modeling intended for a parameter study performed herein.

The effect of liner fixation types on strain energy density in the acetabulum clearly could be demonstrated. The use of a polyethylene insert leads to stress concentrations at the proximal central part of the acetabulum. This fact remains valid for inclined forces up to 40°. Due to the changes in force transmission between insert and metal shell, a ceramic liner leads to a more even distribution of stresses. Inclined loads are transmitted at the direction of the resulting vector. Using a sandwich-type liner causes a ring shaped centralization of the stress distribution. Inclining the resulting load leads to an elliptical deformation of the strain energy density distribution.

The impact of strain energy density on the prediction of implant survival [36,37] as well as on the amount of bone remodeling [38,39] is still under discussion. Nevertheless determination of strain energy distribution is a valid instrument to investigate postoperative conditions of implant load. There have been no efforts whatsoever to investigate strain distribution during the gait cycle as well as changes in strain distribution due to bone remodeling. The simplification of the complex anatomic structures again leads to a more uniform strain distribution. It is assumed that modeling the whole pelvis including muscles and ligaments will effect the strain distribution as well. The simulation of subchondral bone may be valid depending on the operation procedure as well as on the quality of the patients' acetabulum. In general strain energy density will become more distributed due to load transmitting effects of the bone plate. Neglecting micromotion between the implant and the acetabulum again may alter the prediction of implant survival. Strictly speaking, the results presented herein are limited to the well ingrown situation.

In spite of these limitations of the Finite Element-method the use of a ceramic liner results in a broadened load transmission and a minor peak strain. However the effect of the altered load transmission on the clinical situation still remains unclear. In cadaver studies of the normal acetabulum employing a load of 1400 N a C-shaped load transmission zone into the three columns of Os ilium, Os ischium and Os pubis was observed. The use of hemispheric acetabular cups with a flattened pole resulted in a similar pattern of load transmission and was therefore assumed to represent a more natural type of load transmission [40]. Other studies proved that a greater contact zone between the implant and the acetabular bone resulted when fixation was achieved especially in the aequatorial region of a hemispheric implant [41]. In clinical studies the press-fit fixation of a hemispheric cup showed superior results compared to screw fixation alone [42, 43]. The broadened load transmission via the periphery of the implant caused by the use of a ceramic liner therefore may support the load transmission pattern intended for an optimum press-fit fixation [40, 44].

However the prediction of the Finite Element-analysis has to be reviewed under a clinical situation [37, 38]. While qualitative radiological changes will not be detected before a period of five years postoperatively the only predictive clinical parameter with biomechanical relevance is the implant migration [45–47]. The effect of different types of liners within an identical metal-alloy shell on implant migration therefore is currently examined in a prospective-randomized study using the Einbildröntgenanalyse (EBRA) method for assessment of cup migration. First results of this study are presented in this volume [48].

References

1. Smith SE, Harris WH (1997) Total hip arthroplasty performed with insertion of the femoral component with cement and the acetabular component without cement. J Bone Joint Surg Am 79: 1827–1833
2. Snorrason F, Karrholm J (1990) Primary migration of fully-threaded acetabular prostheses. J Bone Joint Surg Br 72: 647–652
3. Yahiro MA, Gantenberg JB, Nelson R et al (1995) Comparison of the results of cemented, porous-ingrowth, and threaded acetabular cup fixation. A meta-analysis of the orthopaedic literature. J Arthroplasty 10: 339–350
4. Harris WH (1993) Keynote address: Clinical considerations. pp. 1–11. In Morrey BF (ed): Biological, material and mechanical considerations of joint replacement. Raven, New York,
5. Schmalzried TP, Kwong LM, Jasty M et al (1992) The mechanism of loosening of cemented acetabular components in total hip arthroplasty. Analysis of specimens retrieved at autopsy. Clin Orthop 274: 60–78
6. Clarke IC, Willmann G (1994) Structural ceramics in orthopedics. pp. 203–252. In Cameron HU (ed.): Bone implants interface, Mosby, St. Louis, Baltimore, Boston
7. Willmann G (1998) Ceramics for total hip replacement – what a surgeon should know. Orthopaedics 21: 173–177
8. Nizard RS, Sedel L, Christel P et al (1992) Ten-year survivorship of cemented ceramic-ceramic total hip prosthesis. Clin Orthop 282: 53–63
9. Heisel J, Mittelmeier H (1993) Medium-term results of cement-free Autophor hip endoprosthesis. Z Orthop 131: 507–12
10. Knahr K, Böhler M, Frank P et al (1987) Survival analysis of an uncemented ceramic acetabular component in total hip replacement. Arch Orthop Trauma Surg 106: 297–300
11. Winter M, Griss P, Scheller G et al (1992) Ten- to 14-year results of a ceramic hip prosthesis. Clin Orthop 282: 73–80
12. Sedel L, Nizard RS, Kerboull L et al (1994) Alumina-alumina hip replacement in patients younger than 50 years old. Clin Orthop 298: 175–183
13. Mahoney OM, Dimon JH (1990) Unsatisfactory results with a ceramic total hip prosthesis. J Bone Joint Surg Am 72: 663–671
14. Böhler M, Knahr K, Plenk H, Jr. et al (1994) Long-term results of uncemented alumina acetabular implants. J Bone Joint Surg Br 76: 53–59
15. Huo MH, Martin RP, Zatorski LE et al (1996) Cementless total hip arthroplasties using ceramic-on-ceramic articulation in young patients. A minimum 5-year follow-up study. J Arthroplasty 11: 673–678
16. Garcia-Cimbrelo E, Martinez-Sayanes JM, Minuesa A et al (1996) Mittelmeier ceramic-ceramic prosthesis after 10 years. J Arthroplasty 11: 773–781
17. Dorlot JM (1992) Long-term effects of alumina components in total hip prostheses. Clin Orthop 282: 47–52
18. Huo MH, Martin RP, Zatorski LE et al (1996) Total hip replacements using the ceramic Mittelmeier prosthesis. Clin Orthop 332: 143–150
19. Snorrason F, Karrholm J, Loewenhielm G et al (1989) Poor fixation of the Mittelmeier hip prosthesis. Acta Orthop Scand 60: 81–85
20. Hyder N, Nevelos AB, Barabas TG (1996) Cementless ceramic hip arthroplasties in patients less than 30 years old. J Arthroplasty 11: 679–686
21. Willmann G, Kalberer H, Pfaff HG (1996) Ceramic acetabulum components for hip endoprostheses. 2: Evaluating design and safety. Biomed Tech Berl 41: 284–290

22 Willmann G (1996) Modularity – the chance to solve the wear problems in total hip replacement. pp. 94–99. In Puhl W (ed): Die Keramikpaarung Biolox in der Hüftendoprothetik, Enke, Stuttgart
23 Blömer W (1997) Design aspects of modular inlay fixation. pp. 95–104. In Puhl, W (ed.): Performance of the wear couple Biolox forte in hip arthroplasty, Enke, Stuttgart
24 Willmann G (1998) Ceramic acetabulum components for hip endoprostheses. 4: Never mix and match. Biomed Tech Berl 43: 184–186
25 Dalla Pria D, Bregant L, Di Marino F (1997) Stiffness of the acetabular cups: A comparative study using the Finite Element method. pp. 136–138. In Puhl, W (ed.): Performance of the wear couple Biolox forte in hip arthroplasty, Enke, Stuttgart
25 Willmann G, Brodbeck A, Effenberger H et al (1998) Investigation of 87 retrieved ceramic femoral heads. pp. 13–18. In Puhl W (ed.): Bioceramics in orthopaedics – new applications, Enke, Stuttgart
26 Riska EB (1993) Ceramic endoprosthesis in total hip arthroplasty. Clin Orthop 297: 87–94
27 Toni A, Sudanese A, Terzi S et al (1997) Ceramic in total hip arthroplasty. pp. 30–33. In Puhl, W (ed.): Performance of the wear couple Biolox forte in hip arthroplasty, Enke, Stuttgart
28 Dalstra M, Huiskes R (1995) Load transfer across the pelvic bone. J Biomech 28: 715–724
29 Pfleiderer M (1997) Mikrobewegung zementfreier Hüftpfannen im Beckenknochen. VDI-Fortschrittsberichte, Reihe 17, Nr. 162, VDI, Düsseldorf
30 Carter DR, Vasu R, Harris WH: Stress distributions in the acetabular region – II. Effects of cement thickness and metal backing of the acetabular component. J Biomech 1: 165–170, 1982
31 Oonoshi H, Isha H, Hasegawa T (1983) Mechanical analysis of the human pelvis and its application to the articular hip joint – by means of the three dimensional finite element method. J Biomech 16: 247–444
32 Dalstra M (1993) Biomechanical aspects of the pelvic bone and design criteria for acetabular prostheses. Dissertation, Nijmegen
33 Rapperport DJ, Carter DR, Schurman DJ (1985) Contact finite element stress analysis of the hip joint. J Orthop Res 3: 435–464
34 Weinans H, Huiskes R, Rietbergen B et al (1993) Adaptive bone remodeling around bonded noncemented total hip arthroplasty: A comparison between animal experiments and computer simulation. J Orthop Res 11: 500–513
35 Levenston ME, Beaupré GS, Schurman DJ, Carter DR (1993) Computer simulation of stress-related bone remodeling around noncemented acetabular components. J Arthroplasty 8: 595–605
36 Turner CH, Anne V, Pidaparti R (1997) A uniform strain criterion for trabecular bone adaptation: Do continuum-level strain gradients drive adaptation? J Biomech 30: 555–563
37 Jacobs CR, Simo JC, Beaupré GS, Carter DR (1997) Adaptive bone remodeling incorporating simultaneous density and anisotropy considerations. J Biomech 30: 603–613
38 Cappello A, Viceconti M, Nanni F, Catania G (1998) Global asymptotic stability of bone remodeling theories: a new approach based on non-linear dynamical system analysis. J Biomech 31: 289–294
39 Lerner AL, Kuhn JL, Hollister SJ (1998) Are regional variations in bone growth related to mechanical stress and strain parameters? J Biomech 31: 327–335
40 Widmer KH, Zurfluh B, Morscher EW (1997) Contact surface and pressure load at implant-bone interface in press-fit cups compared to natural hip joints. Orthopäde 26: 181–189
41 Kwong LM, O'Connor DO, Sedlacek RC et al (1994) A quantitative in vitro assessment of fit and screw fixation on the stability of a cementless hemispherical acetabular component. J Arthroplasty 9: 163–170
42 Schmalzried TP, Harris WH (1992) The Harris-Galante porous-coated acetabular component with screw fixation. J Bone Joint Surg Am 74: 1130–1139
43 Schmalzried TP, Wessinger SJ, Hill GE et al (1994) The Harris-Galante porous acetabular component press-fit without screw fixation. J Arthroplasty 9: 235–242
44 MacKenzie JR, Callaghan JJ, Pedersen DR et al (1994) Areas of contact and extent of gaps with implantation of oversized acetabular components in total hip arthroplasty. Clin Orthop 298: 127–136
45 Krismer M, Stöckl B, Fischer M et al (1996) Early migration predicts late aseptic failure of hip sockets. J Bone Joint Surg Br 78: 422–426
46 Stocks GW, Freeman MAR, Evans SJ (1995) Acetabular cup migration. Prediction of aseptic loosening. J Bone Joint Surg Br 77: 853–861
47 Hendrich C, Bahlmann J, Eulert J (1997) Migration of the uncemented Harris-Galante acetabular cup – results of the Einbildröntgenanalyse (EBRA) method. J Arthroplasty 12: 889–895
48 Hendrich C, Blanke M, Sauer U, Rader CP, Eulert J (2000) Klinische Ergebnisse und Migrationsanalyse – PLASMACUP, pp. 26–34. In Willmann G, Zweymüller K (eds.): Proceedings of the 5th International Symposium, Thieme, Stuttgart

1.12 Acetabular Ceramic Insert Breakage in Total Hip Prostheses

D. Rueda, F. Barahona

Abstract

Alumina ceramics possess superb tribologic characteristics and an exceptional degree of biotolerance but a new complication has arisen when using total hip prostheses with ceramic-ceramic couplings: breakage of the ceramic insert.

Ceramic head breakage is very well documented in the literature but acetabular ceramic insert breakage is much less well-documented.

2 Reliability – Clinical and Technical Aspect

2.1 Einschränkung der Range of Motion von Hüftendoprothesen durch Design, Position und Pfannenabrieb

R. Bader, G. Willmann

Einleitung

Mehr als 500 000 künstliche Hüftgelenke werden heute weltweit pro Jahr implantiert, allein in Deutschland ca. 150 000. Dabei haben sich die modular aufgebauten Systeme klinisch bewährt. Ein modernes, modulares System besteht aus einem Schaft, auf dem ein Kugelkopf aus Metall oder Keramik aufgesteckt wird. Die meist zementfrei zu implantierende Pfanne besteht aus einem Metallgehäuse (metal-back) und einem Pfanneneinsatz (Insert). Es werden Pfanneneinsätze aus Keramik, Metall oder Polyethylen (PE), vereinzelt auch aus Verbundwerkstoffen (Compositen) verwendet. Auf Grund gestiegener Lebenserwartung in der Bevölkerung und erweiterter Indikationsstellung sind längere Standzeiten für Hüftendoprothesen erforderlich. Ursachen eines Prothesenversagens sind meist aseptische Lockerung, seltener Luxation, Infektion und technisches Versagen (Verschleiß bei PE-Pfannen, metallischer Abrieb oder Randabplatzer bei Keramik-Inserts). Für den Langzeiteinsatz haben sich bisher die Gleitpaarungen Keramikkopf/PE-Pfanne mit Abriebraten von unter 0,1 mm/Jahr und die Paarung Keramikkopf/Keramikpfanne mit der Option auf um 0,001 mm/Jahr klinisch bewährt.

Bei der Entwicklung und Realisierung eines Hüftendoprothesensystems sind einige Gesichtspunkte zu beachten. Ein wichtiger Aspekt ist hierbei der Bewegungsumfang des künstlichen Hüftgelenkes, die sogenannte Range of Motion (ROM).

Bei unzureichendem Bewegungsumfang kann der Prothesenhals am Pfannenrand anschlagen (= Impingement). Der auftretende Materialkontakt führt bei Pfannen bzw. Inserts aus PE zu einer Verformung durch Kaltfluss und einem etwas später einsetzenden hohen Verschleiß (Abb. 1), welcher eine durch Partikel induzierte Osteolyse fördert. Auch bei bipolaren Hüftendoprothesen

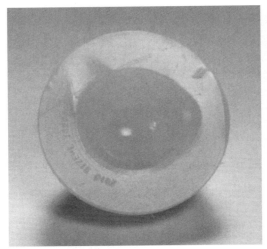

Abb. 1 Verformung einer PE-Pfanne durch Kaltfluss und Abrieb, deutlicher Materialverschleiß am medialen Pfannenrand durch Impingement.

mit PE-Inserts sind osteolytische Prozesse infolge Impingement beschrieben. Durch wiederholtes Anschlagen am Pfannenrand können auch metallische Partikel vom Prothesenhals abgerieben bzw. freigesetzt werden. An keramischen Pfannen(einsätzen) kann ein Impingement Absplitterungen am Rand oder einen Bruch nach sich ziehen (Abb. 2a und 2b). Echte Insertbrüche wurden sehr selten beobachtet, meist handelt es sich um Randabplatzer. Osteolytische Reaktionen infolge keramischer Bruchpartikel sind bisher nicht beschrieben.

Eine bisher relativ wenig beachtete Tatsache ist die Einleitung von Torsionsmomenten in das Interface Knochen – Pfannengehäuse bei Impingement (Abb. 3). Durch Anschlagen des Halses werden Relativbewegungen am Interface ausgelöst, die ab einer gewissen Größenordnung zu einer aseptischen Lockerung der Pfanne führen können.

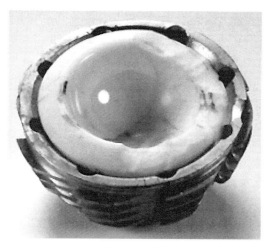

Abb. 2a Abplatzungen am überstehenden Rand des keramischen Pfanneneinsatzes, metallische Abriebspuren des Prothesenhalses am Insertrand.

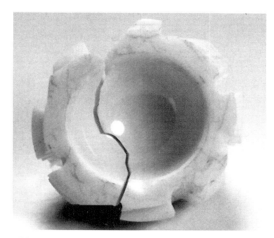

Abb. 2b In vivo Bruch einer monolithischen Keramikpfanne, die heute nicht mehr verwendet wird.

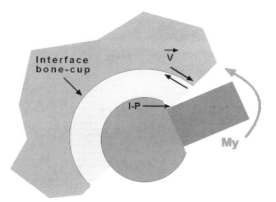

Abb. 3 Einleitung eines Torsionsmomentes (z. B. My bei Abduktion) bei Impingement (I-P = Kontaktpunkt) über die Pfanne ins das Interface Implantat-Knochen mit möglichen Relativbewegungen.

Für den Erfolg einer Hüftendoprothesenoperation und die Zufriedenheit des Patienten ist auch der postoperative Bewegungsspielraum im künstlichen Gelenk in Abhängigkeit vom Aktivitätsgrad höchst relevant. Es erfordern schon alltägliche Bewegungen (wie Strümpfe anziehen, Schuhe zubinden, Benutzung von Verkehrsmitteln etc.) bereits bei weniger aktiven Patienten eine nicht zu unterschätzende ROM. Um ein postoperatives Wohlbefinden erzielen und ein Stück Lebensqualität zurückgewinnen zu können, muss eine ausreichende postoperative Hüftbeweglichkeit des Patienten gewährleistet sein, ein spürbares Anschlagen der Prothese führt hingegen zu einer Verunsicherung des Patienten.

Range of Motion vs. Implantatdesign und –position

Um den Einfluss von Implantatdesign und -stellung auf die ROM von Hüftendoprothesen analysieren zu können, wurden in einem 3D CAD-System die Bewegungsabläufe an Hüftprothesenmodellen bei verschiedenen Implantatpositionen und Prothesendesigns simuliert. Die Untersuchungsergebnisse zeigen die Bedeutung einer korrekten Position der Pfanne und den starken Einfluss von Designmerkmalen der Hüftpfanne, von Prothesenkopfgröße und Konus-Hals-Geometrie auf die ROM, die sich insbesondere bei jungen aktiven Patienten am physiologischen Bewegungsumfang orientieren sollte.

Bei Pfannen mit keramischem Insert (gilt im übrigen auch für Metall- und PE-Inserts) ist eine Inklination von 45° und eine Anteversion (AV) von 15° anzustreben. Bei 30° Inklination ist gegenüber 45° Inklination der Umfang von Flexions-, Extensions- und Abduktionsbewegungen um bis zu 20° eingeschränkt (Abb. **4a**). Bei Steilstellung der Pfanne (z.B. 60° Inklination) steigt die ROM für Flexion, Extension und Abduktion zwar an, jedoch finden sich niedrigere Bewe-

2.1 Einschränkung des Bewegungsumfanges von Hüftendoprothesen

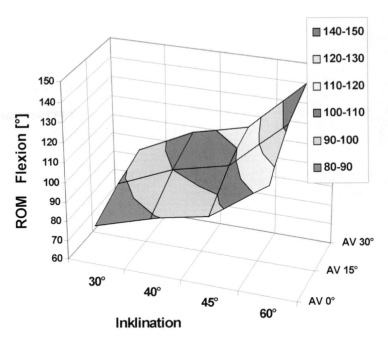

Abb. 4a Einfluss der Pfannenposition auf die ROM für Flexion bei hemisphärischer, randbündiger Pfanne kombiniert mit einem Geradschaft (⌀ 28 mm Kopf, Konus 12/14, CCD-Winkel 135° und Antetorsion 0°).

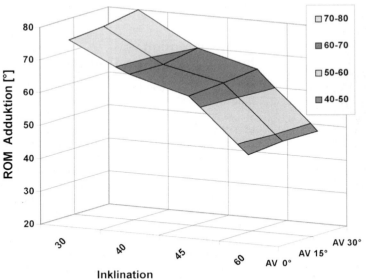

Abb. 4b Einfluss der Pfannenposition auf die ROM für Adduktion bei hemisphärischer, randbündiger Pfanne kombiniert mit einem Geradschaft (⌀ 28 mm Kopf, Konus 12/14, CCD-Winkel 135° und Antetorsion 0°).

gungsumfänge für Adduktion, Außen- und Innenrotation (Abb. **4b**). Eine Innenrotation, kombiniert mit 45° Flexion und 10° Adduktion, ist z. B. nur bis 31° möglich (vs. 40° bei 45° Inklination). Neben dem erhöhten Luxationsrisiko steigt bei steilgestellten Pfannen auch die Gefahr von Randabplatzern bei Keramikinserts infolge erhöhter Hertzscher Flächenpressung am kraniolateralen Pfannenrand an.

Pfannen mit überstehendem Rand des keramischen BIOLOX® Inserts (Abb. **5**), wie sie in der 1. Generation 1986 eingeführt worden sind, soll-

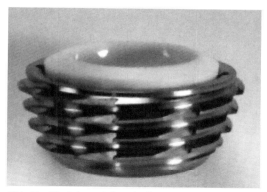

Abb. 5 Modulare Schraubpfanne mit überstehendem Rand des keramischen BIOLOX® Inserts der 1. Generation.

ten wegen erhöhten Risikos von Impingement nicht benutzt werden. Pfannen mit keramischen BIOLOX®forte Einsätzen der 2. Generation, die mit etwas zurückgesetztem Rand ausgerüstet sind, minimieren das Risiko von Impingement deutlich.

Systeme mit randgeschütztem Keramikinsert (durch zusätzlichen PE-Ring) führen im Vergleich zur randbündigen, hemisphärischen Pfanne zu einer massiven Einschränkung der ROM von etwa 20° bis 25°, ein Impingement ist schon bei einfachen alltäglichen Bewegungen höchst wahrscheinlich. Derartige Systeme sollten nicht implantiert werden, da der Bewegungsspielraum des Patienten stark eingeschränkt ist und frühzeitiges Prothesenversagen durch Luxation des Prothesenkopfes oder des PE-Schutzringes nach einem Anschlagen des Prothesenhalses an die Pfanne ausgelöst werden kann.

Daneben sollte die Bedeutung der Randgeometrie der Pfanne bzw. des Inserts auf die ROM der Hüftendoprothese beachtet werden, schon durch geringe konstruktive Veränderungen am Pfannenrand kann sich der Bewegungsumfang erhöhen. Beispielsweise steigert ein Zunahme des Rundungsradius an einem keramischen Pfanneneinsatz (von Radius 0 auf Radius 2,3 mm) die ROM aller Bewegungsformen um etwa 5° (bei hemisphärischer, randbündiger Pfanne mit einem ⌀ 28 mm Kugelkopf und zylindrischem Konus 12/14).

Kopfgröße und Halsdurchmesser bzw. -geometrie haben einen entscheidenden Einfluss auf die ROM einer Hüftendoprothese. Bei Verwendung kleinerer Köpfe ist mit einer Einschränkung der ROM zu rechnen. Im Vergleich zu einem ⌀ 28 mm Kugelkopf mit Konus 12/14 ist bei einem ⌀ 22 12/14 Kugelkopf die ROM um 10° bis 15° eingeschränkt, der Unterschied zwischen ⌀ 28 mm und ⌀ 26 mm beträgt etwa 4° bis 5°. Bei hemisphärischen, randbündigen Pfannen unter einer Inklination von 45° besitzt ein Kugelkopf mit ⌀ 32 mm bzw. mit ⌀ 36 mm gegenüber einem mit ⌀ 28 mm einen um etwa 6° bzw. 10° größeren Bewegungsspielraum für Flexion (bei identischer Konusgeometrie). Die ROM-Erhöhung gilt für alle Bewegungen des künstlichen Hüftgelenkes, deren Ausmaß differiert in Abhängigkeit von Bewegungsform, Inklination bzw. Anteversion der Pfanne und Antetorsion des Schaftes. Mit zunehmender Prothesenkopfgröße steigt zudem die Stabilität des künstlichen Hüftgelenkes gegenüber einer Luxation an.

Eine ⌀ 28 mm Halskugel führt im Vergleich zu einem ⌀ 28 mm Kugelkopf zu einer Einschränkung der ROM um etwa 20°.

Das Verhältnis von Kopf- zu Halsdurchmesser sollte stets ≥ 2 betragen. Zwischen Kugelkopf ⌀ 22 mit Konus 9/11, ⌀ 26 mit Konus 11/13 und ⌀ 28 mit Konus 12/14 finden sich keine nennenswerten Unterschiede im Bewegungsumfang (Abb. 6). Modifikationen an der Geometrie des Prothesenhalses führen zu einer veränderten ROM, z. B. bewirkt eine Hinterschneidung am zylindrischen Hals von 14 mm auf 12 mm eine Erhöhung der ROM um durchschnittlich 7°.

Der CCD-Winkel des Schaftes beeinflusst ebenso die Beweglichkeit der Hüftendoprothese. Bei steigendem CCD-Winkel werden erhöhte Bewegungsumfänge für Abduktions-, Außen- und Innenrotationsbewegungen gemessen, die ROM für Flexion, Extension und Adduktion ist hingegen eingeschränkt. Die ROM für Flexion differiert zwischen dem 125° und 145° Schäften um etwa 20°, d. h. unter 45° Inklination ist bei randbündiger Pfanne mit ⌀ 28 mm Kopf und 125° Schaft eine Flexion bis 106° möglich, bei einem 145° Schaft nur bis 85° (Tab. 1). Nach Möglichkeit sollte der CCD-Winkel des Schaftes nicht über 135° liegen, da bei zunehmenden CCD-Winkel die Luxationstendenz und das biomechanische Risiko (u. a. Zunahme der Hertzschen Flächenpressung am kranio-lateralen Pfannenrand) erhöht sind. Offset bzw. die Kopf-Halslänge der Prothese sollten bereits in der präoperativen Planung Berücksichtigung finden.

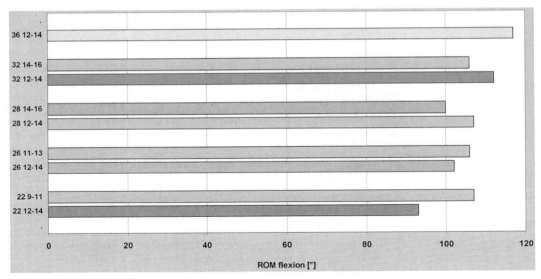

Abb. 6 Einfluss unterschiedlicher Kopf- und Halsdurchmesser auf die ROM für Flexion bei hemisphärischer, randbündiger Pfanne (Inklination 45°, AV 15°) kombiniert mit einem Geradschaft (CCD-Winkel 135° und Antetorsion 0°).

Tab. 1 ROM in Abhängigkeit unterschiedlicher CCD-Winkel des Schaftes (125°, 135°, 145°, jeweils mit ⌀ 28 mm Kopf und Konus 12/14) in Kombination mit einer hemisphärischen, randbündigen Hüftpfanne in 45° Inklination und AV 0°, AV 15°, AV 30°.

	ROM [°] CCD 135°			ROM [°] CCD 125°			ROM [°] CCD 145°			ROM [°] phys.
	AV 0	AV 15	AV 30	AV 0	AV 15	AV 30	AV 0	AV 15	AV 30	
flexion	95	107	114	106	118	121	85	98	106	120–130
extension	95	78	61	106	88	66	85	69	53	20
abduction	63	62	57	52	51	46	73	72	66	30–60
adduction	63	64	65	72	73	74	53	53	54	20–30
ext. rotation	94	80	64	85	70	55	106	92	75	40–50
int. rotation	94	110	125	85	100	119	106	120	133	40–50

Range of Motion vs. Pfannenabrieb

Die Beweglichkeit des künstlichen Hüftgelenkes wird durch Abrieb der Pfanne negativ beeinflusst. Der Prothesenkopf kann infolge von PE-Abrieb in die Pfanne penetrieren, bei der Gleitpaarung Metallkopf mit PE-Pfanne ca. 0,2 bis 0,5 mm pro Jahr, bei Keramikkopf mit PE-Pfanne ca. 0,1 mm pro Jahr. Die jährliche PE-Abriebrate steigt bei Zunahme der Pfanneninklination und der Kopfgröße an. Dagegen scheint die niedrige Abriebrate der Al_2O_3/Al_2O_3 Gleitpaarung (etwa 0,001 mm/Jahr) von der Pfannenposition unbeeinflusst zu sein. Die Folgen einer Penetration des Kopfes sind eine erniedrigte ROM auf Grund eines frühzeitigen Anschlagens des Prothesenhalses am Pfannenrand (Abb. 7) sowie erhöhte Reibmomente an der Grenzfläche Pfanne-Prothesenkopf, die den PE-Abrieb verstärken können. Des Weiteren besteht ein direkter Zusammenhang zwischen Abriebrate und Inzidenz der Pfannenmigration. Die frühzeitige Wanderung (Migration) der Pfanne ist ihrerseits eng mit dem Auftreten einer aseptischen Lockerung verbunden. Der Prothe-

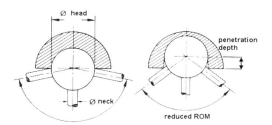

Abb. 7 Einschränkung der ROM nach Penetration des Prothesenkopfes in Richtung Pfannenkuppel (modifizierte Darstellung nach Swanson und Freeman „Die wissenschaftlichen Grundlagen des Gelenkersatzes").

senkopf kann sich bei zunehmender Penetration dezentralisieren, durch die fehlende Übereinstimmung der Drehzentrenposition von Kopf und Pfanne werden Kippmomente induziert. Die Kippmomente können (durch Auslösung von Relativbewegungen) eine aseptische Pfannenlockerung verursachen.

Die Folge einer durch Abrieb verursachten Verlagerung des Prothesenkopfes auf die ROM von Hüftendoprothesen wurde in Abhängigkeit von unterschiedlichen Pfannenpositionen analysiert, indem ein ⌀ 28 mm Kugelkopf, kombiniert mit einem Schaft mit zylindrischem Hals, Konus 12/14, CCD-Winkel von 135°, Schaftantetorsion 0° und einer randbündigen Pfanne, um 0, 1, 2 und 5 mm in Richtung Pfannenkuppel verschoben wurde (Typ A). Da an explantierten PE-Pfannen eine Hauptabriebsrichtung in supero-medialer Richtung von 84° zur Horizontalen (Hall et al. 1998) beschrieben ist, wurde zudem der Prothesenkopf unter diesem Winkel um 0, 1, 2 und 5 mm in die Pfanne verlagert (Typ B). Bei beiden Penetrationsarten wurden die Hüftgelenksbewegungen in 12 verschiedenen Pfannenpositionen (Inklination 30°, 40°, 45°, 60° mit Anteversion 0°, 15°, 30°) ermittelt.

Die Untersuchung zeigt eine deutliche Einschränkung der ROM bei zunehmender Verlagerung des Kopfes. Nach 1 mm Verlagerung ist z. B. die Flexion um etwa 7°, die Abduktion um etwa 4° und Rotationsbewegungen um etwa 7° eingeschränkt, respektive nach 2 mm Verlagerung etwa 15°, 8° und 14°, jeweils bei einem Inklinationswinkel von 45°. Flexionsbewegungen sind bei einer Penetration nach Typ B stärker eingeschränkt (Abb. 8), dies gilt auch für Extension und Abduktion. Falls die Pfanne flacher implantiert wird (z. B. 30° Inklination), werden insbesondere für Flexion niedrige Bewegungsumfänge beobachtet. Nach Verlagerung des Kopfes um 2 mm (entsprechend einer 10-jährigen Laufzeit der Gleitpaarung Metall-PE) ist z. B. bei 30° Inklination und 15° Anteversion der Pfanne die Flexion auf 75° beschränkt. Nach 5 mm Verlagerung findet sich im unserem Modell eine Restriktion der ROM auf 55°, zum Vergleich beträgt die physiologische ROM für Flexion ca. 120°. Bei Steilstellung der Pfanne (z. B. 60° Inklination) steigt die ROM für Flexion, Extension und Abduktion an, jedoch finden sich niedrigere Bewegungsumfänge für Außen- und Innenrotation, beispielsweise ist eine Innenrotation, kombiniert mit 45° Flexion und 10° Adduktion, nach 2 mm Penetration des Kopfes nur noch bis 21° möglich vs. 28° bei einer Inklination von 45°. Dies kann ein erhöhtes Luxationsrisiko nach sich ziehen.

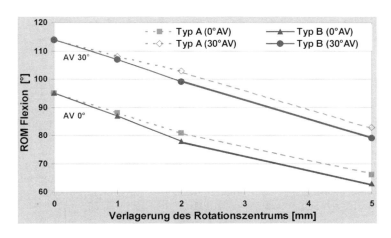

Abb. 8 ROM für Flexion nach Verlagerung des Rotationszentrums vom Prothesenkopf bei 45° Inklination und 0° bzw. 30° Anteversion der Pfanne. Typ A (gestrichelte Linie) Penetration in Richtung Pfannenkuppel, Typ B (durchgezogene Linie) Penetration in supero-medialer Richtung (84° zur Horizontalen).

Range of Motion vs. Luxation

Nach künstlichem Ersatz des Hüftgelenkes ist eine Luxation der Endoprothese eine schwerwiegende Komplikation. Die Inzidenz einer postoperativen Luxation wird zwischen 3% und 5% angegeben, bei Wechseloperationen ist sie deutlich erhöht. Eine Reihe von Risikofaktoren sind beschrieben. Die wichtigsten sind neben dem operativen Zugangsweg ein unzureichendes Implantatdesign sowie eine ungünstige Implantatposition, welche für ca. 30% aller Luxationen verantwortlich gemacht wird.

Für die Auslösung einer Hüftendoprothesenluxation sind nun drei wesentliche Wege beschrieben:
1. Bei Schwäche von Kapsel- und Bandstrukturen bzw. der Hüftmuskulatur (operativ bedingt, neurologische Grunderkrankung etc.) kann der Prothesenkopf ohne ein Impingement über den Pfannenrand gleiten und luxieren.
2. Bei Anschlagen des Prothesenhalses an einem Knochenvorsprung (v.a. an Osteophyten, die intraoperativ nicht beseitigt wurden) kann der Prothesenkopf aus der Pfanne herausgehebelt werden, meist bei einer Überstreckbewegung des Beines.
3. Bei Bewegungen des Beines, welche die ROM der Hüftprothese übersteigen, kann der Prothesenkopf nach Kontakt der Halses am Pfannenrand luxieren (Impingement Prothesenhals-Pfannenrand) (Abb. 9).

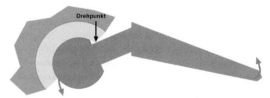

Abb. 9 Luxation des Prothesenkopfes nach Impingement, Kontaktpunkt Pfannenrand-Prothesenhals wirkt als neuer Drehpunkt der Schaftbewegung.

Bei keramischen Pfanneneinsätzen kann es bei einem Impingement, einer Luxation oder Reposition des Kopfes zu einer lokaler Überbeanspruchung des Werkstoffes mit etwaigen Versagen (Randabplatzer oder Bruch) kommen, begünstigt durch eine im Vergleich zu PE geringere Schadenstoleranz.

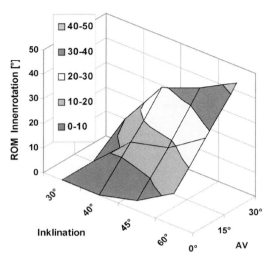

Abb. 10 a ROM für Innenrotation (IR) nach 90° Flexion in Abhängigkeit vom Inklinations- und Anteversionswinkel bei hemisphärischer, randbündiger Pfanne mit ⌀ 32 mm Kugelkopf und Konus 12/14.

Im Simulationsmodell wurden nun der Einfluss von Position und Design der Implantate auf die ROM des künstlichen Hüftgelenkes bei einigen mit einer Luxation assoziierten Bewegungen analysiert. Am Beispiel der Innenrotationsbewegung nach 90° Flexion wird deutlich, dass mit flachgestellter, hemisphärischer, randbündiger Pfanne (30° Inklination) eine ungenügende ROM erzielt wird (Abb. 10 a), ein frühzeitiges Impingement mit Subluxation oder Luxation nach posterior ist möglich. Bei 45° Inklination mit 15° bis 30° Anteversion der Pfanne werden höhere Bewegungsumfange erzielt. Bei Steilstellung der Pfanne (60° Inklination) findet sich jedoch eine zunehmende Einschränkung der ROM für Adduktion, Außen- und Innenrotation, vor allem bei der stark luxationsgefährdeten Bewegung Flexion mit Adduktion und Innenrotation. Generell steigt hier das Luxationsrisiko durch eine geringflächige kraniale Überdachung des Prothesenkopfes durch die Pfanne an. Durch Verwendung von größeren Kugelköpfen kann die Kontaktfläche und die ROM gesteigert werden, beispielsweise ist unter 45° Inklination und 15° Anteversion der Pfanne eine Innenrotation mit 90° Flexion und 10° Adduktion bei dem ⌀ 36 mm 12/14 Kopf bis 19° möglich, bei dem ⌀ 28 mm 12/14 Kopf nur bis 9° (Abb. 10 b).

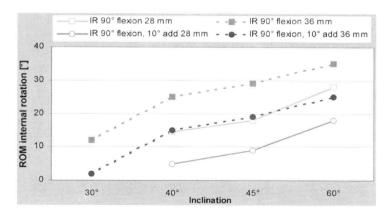

Abb. 10 b ROM für Innenrotation (IR) nach 90° Flexion bzw. 90° Flexion und 10° Adduktion in Abhängigkeit vom Inklinationswinkel bei hemisphärischer, randbündiger Pfanne (AV 15°) und vom Kugelkopfdurchmesser (∅ 28 mm 12/14 vs. ∅ 36 mm 12/14).

Schlussfolgerungen

Moderne Prothesensysteme sollten eine ausreichende Beweglichkeit im künstlichen Hüftgelenk erlauben. Mit Berücksichtigung von konstruktiven, operationstechnischen und tribologischen Randbedingungen kann einem Impingement und einer Luxation wirksam vorgebeugt werden. Konsequenterweise sollten Systeme mit randbündigem Pfanneneinsatz sowie einem Schaft, dessen CCD-Winkel und Halsdurchmesser hinsichtlich ROM auf die übrigen Prothesenkomponenten abgestimmt ist, Verwendung finden. Systeme mit Halskugel oder zusätzlichem PE-Ring zum Schutz des Keramikinserts sollten nach Möglichkeit nicht verwendet werden, da die ROM deutlich eingeschränkt ist. Das Verhältnis von Kopf- zu Halsdurchmesser sollte stets ≥ 2 betragen. Mit zunehmender Prothesenkopfgröße erhöht sich neben dem Bewegungsumfang auch die Stabilität des künstlichen Hüftgelenkes gegenüber einer Luxation, bei Gleitpaarungen mit PE leider auch das Abriebvolumen. Gleitpaarungen mit niedrigen Abriebraten wie die Keramik-Eigenpaarung sollten eingesetzt werden, um Abrieb und Penetration des Kopfes mit frühzeitigem Versagen durch eine PE-Partikel induzierte aseptische Prothesenlockerung zu verhindern; insbesondere bei jüngeren Patienten, bei denen Standzeiten der Hüftendoprothesen von 20 bis 25 Jahren angestrebt werden. Eine exakte intraoperative Positionierung der Implantate ist zu fordern. Als eine ideale Position für Pfannen mit keramischen Inserts sind eine Inklination von 45° und eine Anteversion von 15° anzusehen. Mittels Einsatz von Navigationssystemen und computer-assistierten Operationssystemen (OP-Robotern) werden neben der exakten präoperativen Planung eine anatomisch-biomechanisch präzise Hüftprothesenimplantation ermöglicht, dies ist im besonderen Maße für Wechseloperationen relevant. Verbesserungen der Prozess- und Ergebnisqualität in der Hüftendoprothetik sind zu erwarten.

Empfohlene Literatur

1 Bader R., Willmann G.: Keramische Pfannen für Hüftendoprothesen Teil 6: Pfannendesign, Inklinationswinkel- und Antetorsionswinkel beeinflussen Bewegungsumfang und Impingement. Biomed. Technik 44 (1999) 212–219.
2 Bader R., Willmann G.: Keramische Pfannen für Hüftendoprothesen Teil 7: Wie beeinflussen Lage des Rotationszentrums und CCD-Winkel des Schaftes Range of Motion und Impingement. Biomed. Technik 44 (1999) 345–351.
3 Bader R., Willmann G.: Range of Motion vs. Impingement. Posterpräsentation 5. International CeramTec Symposium, CeraNews Extra (2000) in Druck.
4 Bader R., Willmann G.: Range of Motion vs. Position and Design. Posterpräsentation 5. International CeramTec Symposium, CeraNews Extra (2000) in Druck.
5 Bader R., Willmann G.: Range of Motion vs. Wear. Posterpräsentation 5. International CeramTec Symposium, CeraNews Extra (2000) in Druck.
6 Bader R., Willmann G.: Range of Motion vs. Dislocation. Posterpräsentation 5. International CeramTec Symposium, CeraNews Extra (2000) in Druck.

7 Hall R. M., Siney P., Wroblewski B. M., Unsworth A.: Observations on the direction of wear in Charnley sockets retrieved at revision. J Bone Joint Surg Br 80 (1998) 1067–1072.
8 McCollum D. E., Gray W. J.: Dislocation After Total Hip Arthroplasty. Clin. Orthop. 261 (1990) 159–170.
9 Morrey B. F.: Instability After Total Hip Arthroplasty. Orthopaedic Clinics of North America 23 (1992) 237–248.
10 Wroblewski B. M.: Revision Surgery in Total Hip Arthroplasty. Springer Verlag, London, Berlin, Heidelberg (1990).

2.2 Pre-Operative Planning in THR is a Must

C. Dietschi, D. Buehler

Abstract

Our aim of THR is an anatomical hip reconstruction with acetabular and femoral prostheses. *Pre-operative p*lanning (POP) is most important.

Perquisites for correct offset and lever arms of weight and muscles as well identical leg length. Our POP is presented in an AP and Lateral plane. In the future 3-dimensional planning can give even more information about exact bone-implant contact and local stresses.

For more information see POP home page: www.muggi.com

2.3 Besteht ein Risiko, wenn keramische Kugelköpfe bei Revisionsoperationen auf in situ belassene Schäfte aufgesetzt werden?

Teil 1: Titankonen[1]

G. Willmann, H. G. Richter, J. Richter, E. Steinhauser

Is There a Risk when Using Ceramic Heads on Not-Revised Stems?
Part 1: Titanium Tapers

Abstract

When performing revision surgeries for changing the acetabular component only a well osseointegrated stem mostly will stay in situ. It is common practice that ceramic heads are put on the tapers of stems that are left in situ. Companies that offer ceramic heads state that there may be the risk that the ceramic head may fracture in vivo.

There are no case reports in the literature and there is no consensus on this topic. Therefore some tests have been performed with titanium tapers.

The surface of titanium tapers that were used for testing the burst strength of ceramic heads had been damaged in the laboratory by indentation or by machining grooves. When measuring the burst strength of ceramic heads the strength is decreasing only if there is an elevation caused by the indentation due to very heavy forces. If so the elevations can easily be detected by visual inspection.

Seven retrieved titanium stems have been used to mimic stems that had stayed in situ during revision surgery. When inspecting the tapers of these stems scratches were detected. The burst strength was measured using these 7 stems. All values were according to FDA's recommendations, i.e. no exaggerated risk of failure may be expected.

1. The risk of ceramic fracture seems to be negligible if the surgeon has not detected any damages, except small scratches with no elevation on the titanium taper of a stem left in situ.
2. The risk of scratching a taper during revision surgery is reduced if the surgeon is using the instruments offered to take off a head.
3. The risk of scratching the taper is reduced if the surgeon puts a protection cap on the taper.
4. If the surgeon has any doubt he always has the back up to use a metal head.

Revisionsoperationen

Die Zahl der Wechseloperationen bei TEPs nimmt ständig zu. Oft wird nur die Pfanne gewechselt, der Schaft bleibt in situ, wenn er gut osseointegriert ist. Wegen des nachweislichen geringen Polyethylenabriebes für die Gleitpaarung Keramik/Polyethylen sollte man bei Patienten mit einer hohen Lebenserwartung diese Option nutzen, die Partikel induzierte Osteolyse und aseptische Lockerung zu vermeiden und keramische Kugelköpfe einzusetzen.

Bei einer Revision der Pfanne wird aus operationstechnischen Gründen der Kugelkopf – egal ob aus Metall oder Keramik – abgezogen, wobei die Gefahr der Beschädigung des Schaftkonus besteht. Laboruntersuchungen im eigenen Haus zeigen, dass die Bruchlast eines keramischen Kugelkopfes abnimmt, wenn der metallische Schaftkonus beschädigt (i. a. zerkratzt) ist.

Es existiert hier also ein Risiko, dass die Tragfähigkeit eines wieder aufgesetzten keramischen Kugelkopfes geringer ist. Dieser Themenkomplex und die nötige Risikoeinschätzung sind auf dem 4. Internationalen CeramTec Symposium am 13. März 1999 in Stuttgart ausführlich diskutiert worden. In Kapitel 2 „Reliability – Clinical Aspects" des Tagungsbandes zum 4. Symposium (1) sind Beiträge erfahrener Chirurgen (2,3,4,5) und eine Stellungnahme der CeramTec (6) abgedruckt.

---

[1] Der Beitrag basiert auf der Diplomarbeit von Dipl. Ing. J. Richter

Während die Chirurgen meistens auf einen in situ belassenen Schaft wieder einen keramischen Kugelkopf aufsetzen, warnen CeramTec und die Prothesenfirmen davor.

Ein Konsens, ob auf einen in situ verbleibenden Schaft ein keramischer Kopf aufgesetzt werden darf, besteht nicht.

Es gilt also, diesen Fragenkomplex genauer zu bewerten und durch experimentelle Untersuchungen, für Entscheidungen und Empfehlungen und eine Risikoeinschätzung eine sachliche Basis zu schaffen. Deshalb wurde u. a. im Rahmen einer Diplomarbeit (7) eine Untersuchung an explantierten Titanschäften durchgeführt.

Material und Methode

Die Belastbarkeit (= Bruchlast, Berstlast) von keramischen Köpfen (hier BIOLOX®forte aus der laufenden Produktion, Durchmesser 28 mm) wurde auf unbeschädigten Prüfkonen (12/14) aus Titanlegierung (TiAl6V4) als Referenz bestimmt. Diese Prüfkonen werden benutzt, um bei Veränderungen in der Herstellung von keramischen BIOLOX®forte Kugelköpfen die Bruchlast der Köpfe zu prüfen. Die Spezifikationen der Titankonen und ihr Einfluss auf die Bruchlast sind in (8) beschrieben. Die Bruchlast bzw. Berstlast der keramischen Kugelköpfe wird nach den Empfehlungen der ISO 7206-5 (9) bestimmt (zum Messprinzip siehe Abb. 1).

Um den Einfluss von beschädigten Konen auf das Bruchrisiko in vivo zu studieren, wurden Prüfkonen aus TiAl6V4 Legierung im Labor reproduzierbar beschädigt. Es sollte die Situation bei einer Revision nachgestellt werden. Danach wurde die Bruchlast von keramischen Kugelköpfen aus BIOLOX®forte auf diesen beschädigten Prüfkonen bestimmt.

Als Modell für in situ belassene Schäfte standen 7 Explantate aus Titanlegierung aus der Klinik für Orthopädie und Sportorthopädie der TU München (Dir. Prof. Dr. Gradinger) zur Verfügung. Beschädigungen an den Konen der Explantate konnten durch visuelle Inspektion leicht nachgewiesen werden. Auf diesen 7 Konen wurde ebenfalls die Bruchlast nach ISO 7206-5 bestimmt.

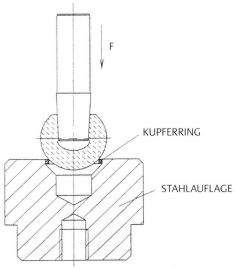

Abb. 1 Aufbau zur Prüfung der Berstlast bzw. Bruchlast keramischer Kugelköpfe nach der Norm ISO 7206-5.

Ergebnisse

Prüfkonen

Im Labor wurden Prüfkonen mit Hilfe des standardisierten und gut reproduzierbaren Methode der Härteprüfung nach Rockwell bzw. Brinell beschädigt (Abb. 2). Außerdem wurden Rillen in die Konen gedrückt. In einigen Fällen führt eine im Labor vorgenommene Beschädigung des Konus zu einer sichtbaren Aufwölbung am Rand, wie z. B. bei einem Eindruck mit dem Härteprüfer (siehe Abb. 3). Diese Aufwölbung entsteht durch die plastische Verformung des Metalls. Bei einem Kratzer auf einem Konus kann dies mit einer Ackerfurche verglichen werden, die ja eine Vertiefung darstellt und am Rand aber einen Aufwurf hat.

Als Kriterium für Sicherheit gegen Versagen werden die Vorgaben der Food and Drug Administration (FDA) genommen. Die FDA gibt Prothesen mit keramischen Kugelköpfen nur frei, wenn auf Originalkonen geprüft, der Mittelwert der Bruchlast der Kugelköpfe nicht unter 46 kN (= ca. 4600 kg) liegt und gleichzeitig keiner der Werte unter 20 kN (= ca. 2000 kg) ist (10).

Nur wenn man bei den im Labor vorgenommenen Beschädigungen eine starke Aufwölbung

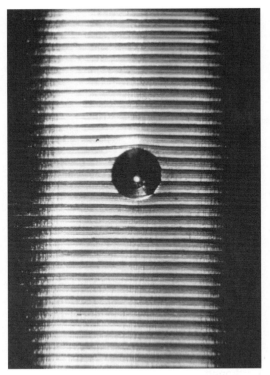

– visuell und mit dem Perthometer – feststellen kann, nimmt die Belastbarkeit des Kopfes ab (siehe die Fälle Nr. 1, 7, 9, und 10 in den Abb. **4a** bzw. **4b**). Die Bruchlasten liegen dann unter den Vorgaben der Food and Drug Administration (FDA).

Verletzungen am Konus, die zu einem erhöhten Versagensrisiko in vivo führen können, werden nach dieser Untersuchung nur mit grober Gewalteinwirkung verursacht. Die Aufwölbung, die wegen der Spannungskonzentration im keramischen Kugelkopf die Ursache für die Abnahme der Bruchlast ist, ist ohne besondere Hilfsmittel gut sichtbar. Der Operateur sollte sie auch im OP problemlos erkennen können.

Explantate

Bei den Bruchlasten auf den 7 explantierten Titanschäften konnten Beschädigungen, wie Kratzer festgestellt werden. Die Beschädigungen konnten durch visuelle Inspektion – ohne Hilfsmittel, also wie sie auch der Chirurg im OP durchführen kann – leicht festgestellt werden. Es wurde nicht, wie erwartet, eine Abnahme der Bruchlast festgestellt (Abb. **5**).

Der Mittelwert der Bruchlasten lag bei 66 kN, der kleinste Wert bei 54 kN und die Standard-

Abb. 2 Beispiel für einen im Labor beschädigten Prüfkonus.

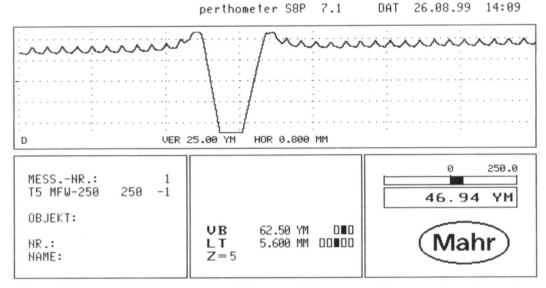

Abb. 3 Prüfkonus aus TiAl6V4 Legierung, beschädigt durch den Eindruck mit einem Härteprüfer. Mit Hilfe des Perthometers kann die Oberflächenstruktur bzw. Rauhigkeit dargestellt werden. Hier sieht man deutlich, dass durch den Eindruck ein Aufwurf entstanden ist.

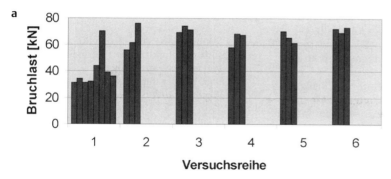

Abb. 4a, b Bruchfestigkeit von keramischen Kugelköpfen aus BIOLOX®*forte*, bestimmt auf beschädigten Prüfkonen aus TiAl6V4 Legierung. Nur wenn die Beschädigung einen Aufwurf aufweist, entspricht die Bruchlast nicht mehr den Vorgaben der FDA, z. B. die Fälle 1, 7, 9 und 10.

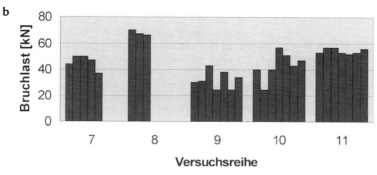

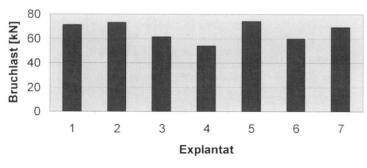

Abb. 5 Die Bruchfestigkeit von keramischen Kugelköpfen aus BIOLOX®*forte*, bestimmt auf den 7 explantierten Titanschäften liegt stets oberhalb 46 kN. Kein Wert liegt unter 20 kN.

abweichung lag bei 7,7 kN. Diese 7 Schäfte hätten als Prüfkonen die Freigabebestimmungen der FDA erfüllt.

Fazit

Auf der Basis dieser (sicher statistisch nicht ausreichend abgesicherten) Studie mit Prüfkonen und 7 Explantaten aus TiAl6V4 Legierung kann man folgern, dass Beschädigungen des metallischen Konus eines Schaftes nur ein Versagensrisiko für einen keramischen Kugelkopf darstellen, wenn sie zu einer deutlich sichtbaren Aufwölbung geführt haben. Diese Aufwölbung ist durch visuelle Inspektion ohne besondere Hilfsmittel leicht festzustellen.

1. Das Risiko der Verletzung des metallischen Konus kann man sicher verringern, wenn man die Abziehinstrumente benutzt, die einige Firmen zur schonenden Entfernung des Kugelkopfes anbieten. Abziehinstrumente für den Kugelkopf vermindern die Gefahr der Verletzung eines Konus deutlich.
2. Während der Revisionsoperation sollte der Konus abgedeckt werden, um zu vermeiden, dass er mit einem Instrument berührt wird. Hierzu stehen Schutzkappen für den Konus zur Verfügung. Sie sollten unbedingt verwendet werden.

3. Der Operateur muss den in situ belassenen Konus vor dem Aufstecken eines Keramikkopfes auf Verletzungen prüfen. Zulässig wären nur kleine Kratzer ohne erkennbaren Aufwurf.

Beachtet man diese Punkte, könnte das Risiko nach Aufsteckens eines Keramikkopfes auf einen in situ belassenen Schaft vertretbar sein, besonders wenn man es zu den klinischen Risiken in Relation setzt, die durch die Entfernung eines fest sitzenden Schaftes entstehen.

Es bleibt offen, ob der Operateur auf Grund seines eingeschränkten Sichtfeldes den Konus hinsichtlich aller relevanten Verletzungen sicher beurteilen kann.

Die letzte Entscheidung und Verantwortung hat immer der Operateur. Schätzt der Operateur das Risiko hoch ein, bleibt ihm immer noch die Möglichkeit, einen Kugelkopf aus Metall aufzusetzen.

Untersuchungen mit Konen aus Kobalt-Chrom-Legierung sind noch nicht abgeschlossen.

Literatur

1 Sedel, L., Willmann, G. (ed.) Reliability and Long-term Results of Ceramics in Orthopaedics. Georg Thieme Verlag, Stuttgart 1999
2 Zweymüller, K. Vorgangsweise und Erfahrungen für den Wechsel keramischer Köpfe. Seite 67–68 in: [1] 1999
3 Griss, P., Clauss, A., Scheller, G. Revisionsstrategie nach Bruch oder Verschleiß von Keramikkomponenten. Seite 69–71 in: Seite 67–68 in: [1] 1999
4 Fröhling, M., Zichner, L., Koch, R. Revisionsstrategie bei der Verwendung von Keramikköpfen. Seite 72–74 in: Seite 67–68 in: [1] 1999
5 Sedel, L. Revision Strategy for Ceramic Implant Failures. Seite 75–76 in: Seite 67–68 in: [1] 1999
6 Willmann, G. CeramTec's Recommendations for Revision when Using BIOLOX forte Femoral Heads. Seite 64–66 in: Seite 67–68 in: [1] 1999
7 Richter, J. Untersuchung der Versagenswahrscheinlichkeit von Kugelköpfen aus BIOLOX®*forte*, die bei einer Revisionsoperation auf in situ belassene Schäfte einer Hüftendoprothese gesetzt werden. Diplomarbeit FH Ulm, 1999
8 Willmann, G. Das Prinzip der Konus – Steckverbindung für keramische Kugelköpfe bei Hüftgelenkprothesen. Mat. – wiss. u. Werkstofftechnik 24 (1993) 315–319
9 ISO 7206–5. Implants for surgery – Partial and total hip joint prostheses – Part 5: Determination of resistance to static load and neck region of stemmed femoral components. ISO 7206–5, 1992
10 Food and Drug Administration (FDA). Guidance Document for the Preparation of Premarket Notification for Ceramic Ball Hip Systems. Food and Drug Administration, Washington D. C. USA, 1995

2.4 Untersuchung von explantierten BIOLOX® Köpfen: Analyse der metallischen Abdrücke in der konischen Bohrung[1]

G. Willmann, A. Brodbeck, H. G. Richter

Retrieved Ceramic BIOLOX® Heads: Investigation of Imprints in the Bore of the Heads

Abstract

The conical bores of 87 retrieved BIOLOX® femoral heads were investigated. When the ceramic femoral head is fixed on a metal taper of the stem, the taper causes an imprint in the bore of a head. The imprint should be a homogenous ring.

In this study it was observed that some of the imprints were not homogenous, they had an asymmetric form. If so there might be the risk that the femoral head might have been loose. Metallosis or fracture might have been caused.

To study this fixing of ceramic heads on titanium tapers was mimicked in the lab. The procedure was
1. positioning the head on the taper,
2. then fixing it with a hammer stroke.

It was observed: When the direction of the stroke that will fix the head was out of the taper axis then the very first metal imprints were asymmetric. Later when the head is loaded (e.g. in vivo with body weight) the head will position itself correctly. If so there is no risk of fracture in vivo or metallosis.

Some of the heads investigated had imprints caused by a metal taper that had a straightness not according to CeramTec's specification. If so this will increase the risk of fracture in vivo.

If the metal taper of the stem has been manufactured and checked according to CeramTec's specification and if the surgeon is fixing the ceramic femoral head according to recommendations there will be no risk of failure.

Problem

Bei der Inspektion von 87 revidierten Kugelköpfen aus BIOLOX® (1) wurden bei einigen der explantierten Köpfe in der konischen Bohrung unsymmetrische Metallabdrücke gefunden.

Dieser Befund könnte bedeuten, dass diese Kugelköpfe nicht fest auf dem Metallkonus des Prothesenschaftes gesessen und eventuell in vivo gewackelt haben. Wenn sich dieser Befund bestätigen würde, dann könnte dies ein großes Risiko z.B. zur Auslösung von Metallose oder Bruch des Kopfes in vivo sein.

Material und Methode

Es standen 87 explantierte, zufällig ausgewählte Kugelköpfe aus BIOLOX® zur Verfügung (1). Diese Köpfe waren aus „alter" Aluminiumoxidkeramik der 1. bzw. 2. Generation, also nicht geHIPte Kugelköpfe (3,6). Leider standen die Schäfte für eine Untersuchung nicht zur Verfügung.

Es handelte sich ausschließlich um BIOLOX® Kugelköpfe mit einem Durchmesser von 32 mm, einem Konus 14/16 (sog. großer Konus). Die Implantate waren bis zu 13 Jahren in vivo (1,8). Die Köpfe haben stets gegen Pfannen aus Polyethylen artikuliert.

Alle Implantate wurden wegen einer Lockerung revidiert. Der Grund für die Revision war nie ein technisches Versagen des Kugelkopfes (1). In (8) wurde bereits über die Untersuchung der Oberfläche dieser Kugelköpfe berichtet. Es konnte bei keinem der Kugelköpfe eine Veränderung der Oberfläche festgestellt werden.

---

[1] Die Arbeit basiert auf Teilen der Diplomarbeit von Achim Brodbeck, die er unter Betreuung von PD Dr. G. Willmann im Werk Plochingen der CeramTec angefertigt hat.

In (10) wurde über den erwarteten Festigkeitsabfall durch Materialermüdung berichtet. Die Untersuchung hat ergeben, dass die Kugelköpfe in vivo stets so belastet (1,8) worden sind, dass die Lasten bzw. Spannungsintensitäten unterhalb der Dauerfestigkeit bzw. Fatigue Limit KIo lag. Es ist also keine Materialermüdung aufgetreten, damit auch kein erhöhtes in vivo Versagensrisiko (10).

Befund

Hier soll nur über die Untersuchung des metallischen Abdruckes in der Bohrung der keramischen Kugelköpfe berichtet werden (1).

Die konische Bohrung in den Kugelköpfen wurde visuell und mit Lichtmikroskop auf Verschleiß, Korrosion und Metallspuren (Metallabdruck im Bereich der Bohrung) inspiziert. Außerdem wurden die Köpfe und die Bohrung vermessen und die Ergebnisse mit den bei der Auslieferung von Feldmühle (heute CeramTec) dokumentierten Maßen in den Protokollen der Fertigung und Qualitätskontrolle verglichen.

Alle Explantate entsprachen in den Maßen den damals gültigen Spezifikationen. Es wurde kein Hinweis auf Verschleiß, Korrosion oder Frettingkorrosion im Bereich der konischen Bohrung der BIOLOX®-Explantate gefunden.

Im Bereich der konischen Bohrung wurde unterschiedliche, metallische Abdrücke gefunden. Abb. 1 zeigt schematisch den Abdruck, der in 32 Fällen (37%) gefunden wurde und der als „normal" (Typ 1), also im Sinne der Konstruktion und Funktion der Konussteckverbindung (2,5) erwartet wird. Abb. 2 zeigt, wie ein derartiger metallischer Abdruck entsteht. Die Oberflächenstruktur auf dem metallischen Zapfen wird plastisch unter der Last verformt und plattet sich ab. Ist der Kugelkopf gut fixiert, entsteht eine ringförmige Berührungsfläche am schmaleren (oberen) Ende des Konus. Durch die hohe Reibung ist der Kopf gut und sicher fixiert (5).

Bei einigen der untersuchten Kugelköpfe wurde eine Abweichung von dieser idealen Abdruckform, wie in Abb. 1 und 2 gezeigt, gefunden. Z.B. zeigt Abb. 3 einen Abdruck (Typ 2) der bei 8 Köpfen (9% der Fälle) beobachtet worden ist. Es wird vermutet, dass der Kugelkopf vom Operateur nur

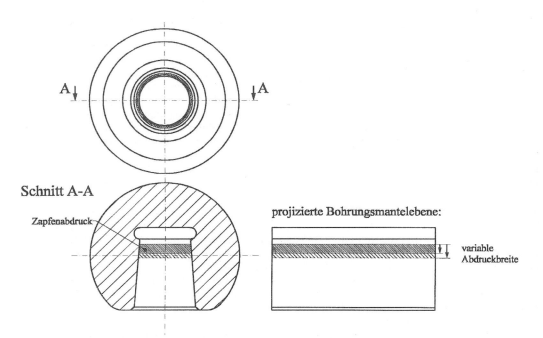

Abb. 1 Abdruck des metallischen Konus eines Prothesenschaftes in der Bohrung von einem explantierten BIOLOX® Kugelkopfes. Abdruck Typ 1 („normal"), gefunden bei 32 der untersuchten Kugelköpfe (37% der untersuchten Fälle).

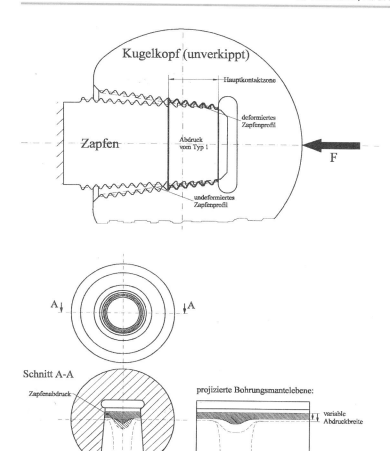

Abb. 2 Verhältnisse bei der Entstehung eines Abdruckes nach Typ 1 („normal").

Abb. 3 Bei 8 Kugelköpfen in dieser Studie wurde ein einseitig asymmetrischer Abdruck (Typ 2) gefunden.

aufgesteckt worden und danach nicht vom Operateur mit einem Einschläger fixiert worden ist.

Abb. 4 zeigt die physiologisch auftretenden Lasten, die i. a. nicht in der Symmetrieachse des Metallkonus liegen. Folgendes wäre vorstellbar: Durch das schräge Aufschlagen auf den Kugelkopf könnte der Kopf zuerst schräg zur Achse des Konus aufsitzen. Durch die ersten Belastungen des Patienten würde er dann zentriert. Es entsteht dann der in Abb. 5 skizzierte metallische Abdruck.

Betrachtet man die physiologisch auftretenden Richtungen der Lasten (Abb. 4), dann drängt sich die Vermutung auf, daß diese keineswegs in der Symmetrierichtung des Konus liegenden Lasten bei einem nicht fest auf dem metallischen Konus fixierten Kopf durch die ständig wechselnden Richtungen der Lasten bei den üblichen Bewegungen zum „Wackeln" des Kopfes führen können. Wie die Erfahrung zeigt, ist dies offensichtlich nicht der Fall, aber es gilt hier eine plausible Erklärung zu finden.

Abb. 6 zeigt einen Abdruck (Typ 3), bei dem der metallische Konus in der Bohrung des Kopfes sowohl am „oberen" (also am Bereich mit dem kleineren Durchmesser), als auch am „unteren" (am Bereich mit dem größeren Durchmesser) Kontakt hatte. Dies wurde in 6 Fällen (7%) beobachtet. Hier gibt es drei Möglichkeiten, wie der Abdruck vom Typ 3 entstanden sein könnte. Abb. 7 zeigt diese Möglichkeiten schematisch auf.

Links oben in Abb. 7 ist der Fall skizziert, daß die Geradheit des metallischen Schaftkonus nicht gemäß den Spezifikationen (2, 5) war. Der metallische Konus ist konkav. Es entsteht so ein Abdruck am oberen und unteren Ende der Bohrung im Kopf. Fest steht, daß bei den 6 Fällen jeweils

2.4 Untersuchung von explantierten BIOLOX-Köpfen: Analyse der metalischen Abdrücke

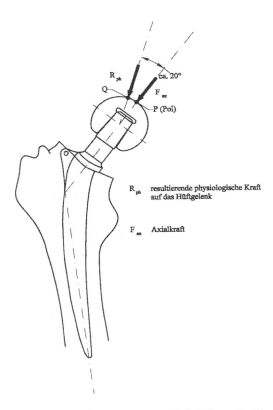

Abb. 4 Lasteinleitung in einen Schaft (schematisch).

der metallische Konus nicht gemäß den Spezifikationen der CeramTec hergestellt worden ist. Es besteht ein erhöhtes Versagensrisiko.

Rechts oben in Abb. 7 ist der Fall skizziert, dass die Bohrung des BIOLOX® Kopfes nicht den Spezifikationen bezüglich der Geradheit entsprach. Dieser Fall kann für diese Untersuchung (1) ausgeschlossen werden, da ja die explantierten BIOLOX® Kugelköpfe alle neu vermessen werden konnten. Sie waren allen gemäß der gültigen Spezifikationen. Es würde ein Abdruck, wie beobachtet entstehen. Aus Untersuchungen an Kugelköpfen anderer Hersteller ist aber bekannt, dass ein derartiger Fall in der Praxis auftreten kann.

Der in Abb. 7 unten skizzierte Fall zeigt die prinzipielle Möglichkeit, dass Kopf und metallischer Konus von den Spezifikationen abweichen.

Es gilt nun zu widerlegen, dass diese Kugelköpfe, die einen Abdruck von Typ 2 aufzeigen, nicht ausreichend auf dem Konus oder „schief" fixiert gewesen wären und in vivo gewackelt hätten.

Hypothese

Das Konzept der Konussteckverbindung setzt voraus, dass alle Lasten vom metallischen Konus (Zapfen) auf die Fläche in der Bohrung des keramischen Kugelkopfes gleichmäßig verteilt eingeleitet werden (2,5). Wenn das so ist, wird ein ringförmiger, gleichmäßig ausgebildeter metallischer Abdruck erwartet (Abb. 1 und 2). Abweichungen würden zu Spannungsspitzen in der Keramik führen (2,5,7,10), die wegen der hohen Sprödigkeit nicht durch Verformung abgebaut werden können. Die Folge ist ein erhöhtes Versagensrisiko durch Bruch ohne Vorwarnung.

Die Kugelköpfe werden vom Operator mit einer Kraft von 1 kN (ca. 100 kg) bis 5 kN (ca. 500 kg) fixiert. Im allgemeinen ist die vom Operateur aufgebrachte Kraft hierbei geringer als die

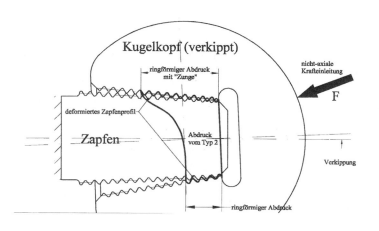

Abb. 5 Vermutete Verhältnisse bei der Entstehung eines Abdruckes vom Typ 2.

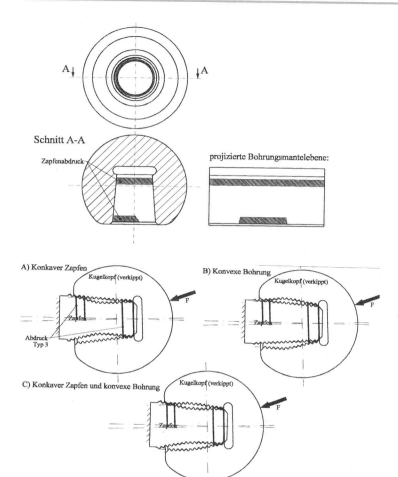

Abb. 6 Abdruck Typ 3 (nicht erwünschter Fall), gefunden in 6 Fällen (7%). Hier hat offensichtlich der metallische Konus die Bohrung sowohl am „oberen" als auch „unteren" Ende berührt.

Abb. 7 Drei Möglichkeiten, wie bei nicht gemäß den Spezifikationen hergestelltem Schaftkonus der Abdruck vom Typ 3 (nicht erwünschter Fall) entstanden sein könnte.

in vivo aufgebrachten Lasten, die ja bekanntlich zwischen dem 3fachen bis 8fachen Körpergewicht (3 kN bzw. ca. 300 kg und 8 kN bzw. ca. 800 kg) liegen. Oft fixierte der Operator den Kugelkopf nicht nach dem Aufstecken des Kopfes auf den Schaftkonus. Oft schlägt der Operator auf den Kugelkopf nicht mit einem Schlag, sondern mit mehreren.

Wichtig ist aber folgendes: Die klinische Erfahrung und Beobachtung ist, **dass der Operateur** nach dem Aufstecken eines Kugelkopfes auf den Konus des Prothesenschaftes bei der anschließenden Fixierung durch einen Schlag mit dem Einschläger **nie genau auf den Kopf in Achsrichtung auf den Konus des Prothesenschaftes aufschlägt.** Dies könnte die Erklärung für die unsymmetrischen metallischen Abdrücke sein.

Modellversuch

Wie die Beobachtung im OP zeigt, erfolgen mehrmalige Aufschläge auf einen Kugelkopf nie aus der gleichen Richtung, sie sind weder in ihrer Intensität gleich, noch in Richtung zu Symmetrieachse des Konus. Mit einem Modellversuch (Abb. **6** oben) kann man die Metallabdrucke in der Keramik, wie bei den Explantaten beobachtet (Abb. **8** unten), nachstellen.

Deshalb wurde folgender Modellversuch durchgeführt:
1. Metallkonen aus TiAl6V4, wie sie zum Prüfen der Berstlast nach ISO 7205-6 verwendet werden, wurden in einem Schraubstock eingespannt.
2. Keramikköpfe wurden von Hand aufgesteckt.

2.4 Untersuchung von explantierten BIOLOX-Köpfen: Analyse der metalischen Abdrücke

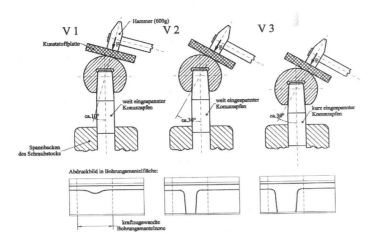

Abb. 8 Modellversuch zum Fixieren eines Kugelkopfes auf einem Konus. *Oben:* Lasteinleitung nicht in Richtung der Symmetrieachse des Schaftkonus. *Unten:* Abdruckbild am oberen Ende der Bohrung des Kugelkopfes. Je größer die Abweichung von der Richtung der Symmetrieachse ist, desto größer ist der metallische Abdruck.

3. Die Keramikköpfe wurden dann schräg zur Symmetrieachse aufgeschlagen (Abb. **8**).
4. Die Richtung des Aufschlages wurde variiert (Abb. **8** oben).

Der Modellversuch zum Fixieren eines Kugelkopfes auf einem Konus zeigt (Abb. **8** unten) das Abdruckbild am oberen Ende der Bohrung des Kugelkopfes. Je größer die Abweichung von der Richtung der Symmetrieachse ist, desto länger und größer ist der metallische Abdruck. Diese Versuche stimmen mit den bei den Explantaten gefundenen Ergebnissen überein.

Es wird von CeramTec in der sog. OP-Chart empfohlen (9), den Kugelkopf vor dem Fixieren mit dem Einschläger mit einer leichten Drehung auf den Konus zu stecken.

Wird der Kopf mit gleichzeitiger leichter Drehung aufgesteckt, zentriert er sich sofort und es entsteht nur ein ringförmiger Abdruck. Oft sitzt der Kugelkopf jetzt schon, ohne dass er mit einem Schlag zusätzlich fixiert worden ist, so fest, dass man ihn nur schwer abziehen kann.

Empfehlung zum Fixieren eines Kugelkopfes

Die folgenden Empfehlungen sind in CeramTec's OP-Chart (9) zusammengestellt. Von Fa. PROTEK ist bereits 1992 in (4) eine ähnliche Empfehlung publiziert worden.
1. Vor Aufstecken eines BIOLOX®*forte* Kugelkopfes ist der Konus des Prothesenschaftes zu reinigen, zu spülen und zu trocken.
2. Der Kugelkopf sollte mit gleichzeitiger leichter Drehung auf den Konus aufgesteckt werden. Dann zentriert der Kugelkopf sich sofort selbst.
3. Ein Schlag mit dem Einschläger zum guten Fixieren des Kugelkopfes auf dem Konus des Schaftes ist ausreichend, mehrere sind zulässig.

Schlussbetrachtung

Man konnte bei den im Labor durchgeführten Modellversuchen alle Metallabdrücke, die man bei den explantierten BIOLOX® Kugelköpfen beobachtet hat (Typ 1 und 2), nachstellen.

Die Versuche zeigen, dass ein Kugelkopf aus BIOLOX®*forte* auf dem Schaftkonus fest und sicher sitzt,
1. wenn der Schaftkonus gemäß den Richtlinien der CeramTec hergestellt und geprüft worden ist;
2. wird der Kugelkopf, wie empfohlen (4,9), aufgesetzt und fixiert, dann ist die Gefahr eines technischen Versagens des Kugelkopfes praktisch ausgeschlossen, wie die klinische Erfahrung mit BIOLOX®*forte* zeigt (3,9).

Literatur

1 Brodbeck A (1997) Risikobewertung von BIOLOX bzw. BIOLOX forte (keramischen) Kugelköpfen für Hüftendoprothesen. Diplomarbeit, Inst. f. Biomed. Technik, Universität Stuttgart

2. Heimke G (1993) Safety Aspects of the Fixation of Ceramic Balls on Metal Stems. Bioceramics 6: 283–288
3. Heros R, Willmann G (1998) Ceramics in Total Hip Arthroplasty: History, Mechanical Properties, Clinical results and Current Manufacturing State of the Art. Seminars of Arthroplasty 9: 114–122
4. PROTEK (1992) BIOLOX – Hüftprothesenköpfe aus Al2O3-Keramik – Wichtige Information für das OP-Team. OP-Journal 8: 102–103
5. Willmann, G (1993) Das Prinzip der Konus-Steckverbindung für keramische Kugelköpfe bei Hüftgelenkprothesen. Mat. wiss. u. Werkstofftechnik 24: 315–319
6. Willmann G, Pfaff HG, Richter H (1995) Steigerung der Sicherheit von keramischen Kugelköpfen für Hüftendoprothesen. Biomed Technik 40: 342–346
7. Willmann, G. (1996) Wie sicher sind keramische Kugelköpfe für Hüftendoprothesen? Mat. wiss. u. Werkstofftechnik 27: 280–286
8. Willmann G, Brodbeck A, Effenberger H, Mauch C, Dalla Pria P (1998) Investigation of 87 Retrieved Ceramic Femoral Heads. In: Puhl W (1998) Bioceramics in Orthopaedics – New Applications. Enke Verlag, Stuttgart, 13–18
9. Willmann G (1999) CeramTec's Recommendations for Revision when Using BIOLOX forte Femoral Heads. In: Sedel L, Willmann G (1999) Reliability and Long-term Results of Ceramics in Orthopaedics. Georg Thieme Verlag, Stuttgart, 64–66
10. Willmann G (1998) Überlebenswahrscheinlichkeit und Sicherheit von keramischen Kugelköpfen für Hüftendoprothesen. Mat. wiss. u. Werkstofftechnik 29: 595–604

2.5 The Status and Early Results of Modern Ceramic-Ceramic Total Hip Replacement in the United States

J. P. Garino

Introduction

Alternate bearing technology has become a significant interest in the United States as many manufacturers are developing programs for this type of technology, including systems of metal/metal, cross-linked poly, and ceramic on ceramic. The reason for such activity in this area is the continued problem of wear and osteolysis of polyethylene, often creating significant challenges at the time of revision due to substantial bone stock depletion.

Alternate bearing technology, at least in concept, is not particularly new. In fact, alternate bearings have been in use for over 25 years, dating back to the mid 60's and early 70's. As we have now entered a new millennium the question can be asked why has the United States lagged in the acceptance and embracing of this new technology compared to our colleagues in other parts of the world. I believe it has to do with the perceptions and misconceptions of American surgeons in general as well as of the FDA and its role in device approval. A better understanding of our current situation can be provided with a brief review of the past.

The initial bearing surface used by Charnley, PTFE, resulted in accelerated wear and suboptimal results. The failure of this material and fears of failure of its replacement material, polyethylene, fueled the alternative bearing development movement. This begun in the 1960's by McKee (1) and others, and in 1970 Pierre Boutin (2) began the ceramic/ceramic era of total hip replacement. The perception in the United States at that time after some early results were available is that the alternate bearing total hip replacements were plagued by poor fixation and no substantial improvement over the metal/polyethylene counterpart could be appreciated. Unlike PTFE, polyethylene had proven itself at least early on to be quite successful. John Charnley and his techniques for the most part were fairly embraced within the United States creating in many ways almost a cult following of his principles.

In 1976, the FDA began device regulation. In the mid 1970's Mittelmeier developed a cementless ceramic/ceramic total hip replacement design. This subsequently came to the United States in the mid 1980's as the Autophor. The Autophor had a number of design flaws, including a monoblock ceramic cup that was screwed into the pelvis. The instrumentation available for inserting it was crude and it was a technically difficult task to properly position the cup within the pelvis. The ball came in skirted varieties, so ceramic/ceramic impingement was not uncommon. This is particularly true following migration and shifting of the cup. The cementless stem did not have any surface texturing or coating supplied and aseptic loosening was commonplace. Rates of poor success in the United States with the Autophor device began to appear in the late 1980's. United States surgeons, for the most part, did not see through these design flaws. They did not fully understand the etiology of these component failures at the time, and, as a result, the ceramic/ceramic couple was implicated.

Polyethylene later emerged as the main culprit in wear debris generation and a subsequent creation of osteolysis (3). With that, a surge in activity in alternate bearings, both within the United States and abroad, began. Enhanced understanding of ceramic biomechanics and biomaterials, particularly that of ceramic quality and taper technology renewed the interest in the ceramic/ceramic couple around the world and eventually in the United States (4). Reports of ceramic fractures, although infrequent and with occurrence essentially limited to poorer quality early ceramic components (5), the concept of fracture remained a significant theoretical problem for American surgeons. Ceramic quality improved with enhanced purity, isostatic pressing

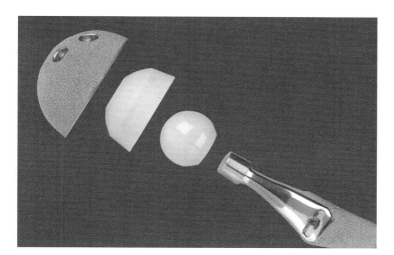

Fig. 1 Modern Ceramic-ceramic THR. Photo courtesy of Smith and Nephew, Memphis, Tennessee, USA.

which reduced the grain size and subsequently, with proof testing, another more consistent level of quality control was initiated, reducing the possibility of ball head fractures even further. Nonetheless, the possibility of a ball head fracture remains a significant concern for American surgeons in general primarily due to the medical legal environment. This is in spite of the fact that ball head fractures have been reduced to approximately to 4 out of every 100,000 for the current state of the art ceramic pieces (6). This compares favorably with any other type of mechanical failure of prosthetic devices.

Modularity of both the head and liner have also contributed greatly to the early success of ceramic bearings and the theoretical high expectations for the long-term survivorship of these devices as fixation and bearing functions are completely separated and optimized.

The Investigational Device Exemption

The development of ceramic on ceramic programs in total hip replacement within the United States lead to examination of these devices by the FDA and this required a classification by the FDA. The ceramic liners, which were really the only new addition to the foray as ceramic ball heads had been approved 10 years previously, and the lack of information regarding these inserts lead the FDA to classify them as a Class 3 device. This high classification resulted in the need for manufacturers to submit a Pre-Market Approval application (PMA) and the bulk of the application would revolve around not only standard laboratory data, but also heavily on clinical data. This clinical data would be collected in the form of an Investigational Device Exemption (IDE), which is a clinical trial performed by the manufacturer with FDA input and support. This is a 4–6 year process which is quite expensive, but nonetheless, with the role and demand for alternate bearings becoming stronger, the manufacturers realizing their potential, began to develop and invest in such programs. As of the winter of the year 2000, the United States IDE's consist primarily of 6 companies. Osteonics and Wright Medical Technology completed their IDE's at least with respect to the initial enrollment groups in the middle portion of 1998. With respect to these two companies it is anticipated that the main cohorts will reach the necessary two year minimum requirement by the FDA later this year. The pre-market approval application will be filed soon thereafter with anticipated approval by the FDA for both companies within the next 12 or so months. Encore Orthopaedics and Smith & Nephew Richards were the next two companies to obtain an approved IDE with these two companies coming on line in late 1998 and early 1999 respectively. Very early in data collection and patient enrollment are Implex and Zimmer and most other manufacturers are developing a program either for the subsequent starting of an IDE or to be poised and ready to move their program to market as soon as this technology is down classified. This usually occurs after three or four

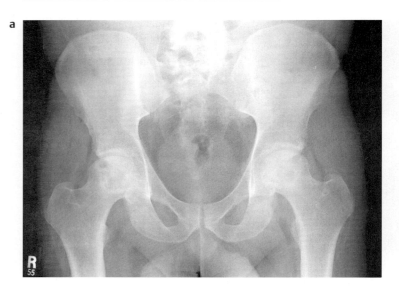

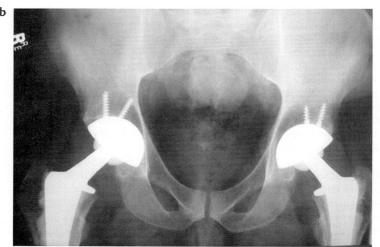

Fig. 2a–d Pre-op (**a**) and 2 year Post-op (**b–d**) of a 38 y/o man with AVN of both hips and collapse.

pre-market approval applications have been endorsed by the FDA.

Data is available regarding the original cohort enrolled in 10 centers, sponsored by Wright Medical Technology. Three hundred thirty patients were enrolled for 1997–1998, 252 of which are now at the minimum two-year follow-up. The average age of these 252 patients is 52 with a range of 25–80. There are 152 males and 100 females. The body mass index averaged at 30 with a range of 18–68.

Diagnoses included osteoarthritis in 162 patients, avascular necrosis in 60, developmental dysplasia in 18, and traumatic arthritis in 11.

Results

The average Harris Hip Score increased from 44 to 97. The average physical portion of the S of 12 increased from 30 to 48. The average mental portion increased from 50 to 56.

There were 27 complications, 5 of which were systemic related and included a myocardial infarction and a pneumonitis. There were 22 hip related complications, including 3 dislocations, 3 calcar or trochanteric fractures intraoperatively, 1 foot drop, 2 superficial infections, 1 deep infection, and 7 various others, including pain and bursitis. There were 4 complications related to

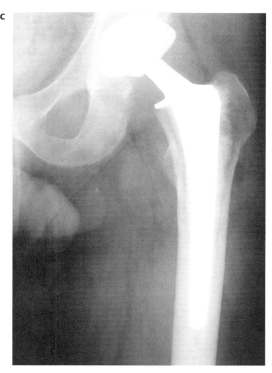

the ceramic pieces, specifically 3 chipped liners and 1 eccentric seating. At the current time, 4 revisions had been performed. One for dislocation anteriorly, one for migration of an acetabular component approximately six weeks after implantation, one for deep infection, and one for eccentric liner placement, which was detected in the recovery room and revised immediately thereafter. These early results compare very favorably with many other series in the literature and represents what might be expected at this early stage with almost any hip replacement system. Of note in the United States, there are well over a thousand patients enrolled in IDE's of one company or another and to date there have been no fractures of ceramic pieces.

Summary

In summary, ceramic bearings are at an investigational stage in the United States. Trials are continuing to go well without problems of fracture. Some designs may even become approved and subsequently available for common use within the United States in approximately one year.

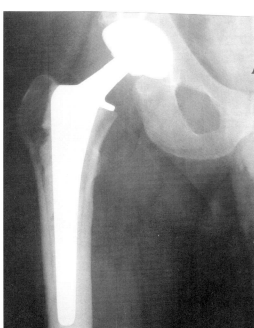

Fig. 2

References

1. McKee GK, Watson-Farrar J: Replacement of the arthritic hips by McKee-Farrar prosthesis. J Bone Joint Surg 48B: 245–259, 1966
2. Boutin PM: Arhroplastic Total de hanche par prosthese en alumine fritte. Rev Chi Orthop 58: 229–246, 1972
3. Schmalzried TP, Jasty M, Harris WH: Periprosthetic bone loss in total hip arthroplasty: role of polyethylene wear debris and the concept of the effected joint space. JBJS 74 A: 849–863, 1992
4. Sedel L, Bizot P., Nizard R, Meunier A. Perspective on a 25 year experience with Ceramic on Ceramic total hip replacement. Seminars in Arthroplasty 9: 123–134, 1998
5. Prudhommeaux F, Nevelos J, Doyle, Meunier A, Sedel L: Analysis of wear Behavior of Alumina-Alumina Hip Prosthesis after 10 years of Implantation. In: Laurent Sedel, Gerd Willmann (Eds): Reliability and Long-term Results of Ceramics in Orthopaedics. Georg Thieme Verlag, Stuttgart, 1999, 111
6. Heros RJ, Wilmann G: Ceramincs in Total Hip Arthroplasty: History, Mechanical Properties, Clinical Results, an Current Manufacturing State of the Art. Seminars in Arthroplasty 9: 114–122, 1998

3 Ion Release Hypersensitivity Allergic Reactions: A Problem in THR?

3.1 Hypersensitivity in THR: A Case Study

E. Seeber

Die Interaktion von Gewebe und Implantat wird von verschiedenen Faktoren bestimmt, u.a. von der metallischen Zusammensetzung der Implantatbestandteile.

Nach der Implantation eines Gelenkersatzes beginnt bewegungs- und belastungsabhängig sofort ein Verschleiß im Bereich der Gleitpaarungen mit Freisetzung eines Abriebs. Die Abriebrate hängt wesentlich vom Gleitpartner z.B. Polyethylen (19) ab in unterschiedlicher Größenordnung je nach primärem Gleitpartner. Dieser kann z.B. aus CoCrMo-Legierungen, CoNiCrMo-Legierung oder Aluminiumoxid bestehen. Die beiden zuletzt genannten werden auch für Gleitflächen mit sich selbst verwendet. Eine Renaissance der sogenannten „harten" Selbstpaarungen wurde insbesondere für das historische Konzept der Metall-Metall-Paarung erwartet (16). Untersuchungen von W. Plitz et al. (13) stellten am Simulationsversuch nach 1,9 Mio. Zyklen Rundheitsabweichungen am Kopf einer Metall-Metall-Paarung mit einem nadelförmigen Belag aus Co, Al, Cl und O fest, dem eine abrasive Eigenschaft zuerkannt wurde.

Die Frage der Immunantwort auf solche Abriebpartikel aus CoCr stellten Merrit et al. (10).

Dagegen untersuchten Jacobs et al. (9) u.a. die CoCr-Konzentration im Urin und Serum, wobei eine toxikologische Interpretation der gefundenen Werte nicht vollzogen wurde.

Seit Mitte der 60er Jahre werden wegen der starken Sensibilisierung durch Allergieprobleme der Bevölkerung zunehmend Titan und Titanlegierungen (6) wegen der Körperverträglichkeit, Korrosionsbeständigkeit und Dauerschwingfestigkeit bei orthopädischen Dauerimplantaten verwendet. Die Verschleißbeständigkeit der Titanlegierungen als Gleitflächenersatz ist jedoch ungenügend. Deshalb kommen Gleitflächen auf Cobalt-Chrom-Basis mit einer Zusammensetzung aus ca. 63% Cobalt, 28% Chrom, 6% Mangan und maximal 1% Nickel (6) noch häufig, überwiegend in der Knieendoprothetik, zur Anwendung. In Schmiedestahl-Prothesen können die Nickel-Konzentrationen zwischen 8,5–14%, die Chromanteile bei 20% liegen (7). Es liegt aber bei ca. 20% der jüngeren weiblichen Bevölkerung eine Nickelallergie vor (18).

Es ist bekannt, dass mit dem niedrigen Nickelgehalt von maximal 1% keine Sensibilisierung eines Patienten aufgebaut werden kann. Besteht aber bereits eine Sensibilisierung, kann je nach patientenspezifischem Reaktionspotenzial selbst diese geringe Menge unerwünschte Gewebsreaktionen (6) induzieren. Außerdem sind die Werkstoffe Cobalt und Chrom ebenfalls allergisierend (11).

Epikutantests mit Chrom, Nickel, Cobalt, metal rust und Endoprothesenspänen ergaben nach Milavec, Puretic et al. (12) bei 9 von 40 Patienten positive Reaktionen, während die induzierte Sensibilisierung durch Metallegierungen bei Metall-Metall-Hüftprothesen von Benson et al. (1) bei 28–46% der Patienten mit Prothesenlockerung beschrieben wird.

Caciller et al. (2) stellte bei 15% der Patienten mit Hüftgelenksersatz eine Metallallergie fest und bei einem von 12 Patienten mit einer aseptischen Lockerung. Eine Allergie auf die plastische Komponente der Implantate ist sehr selten (3, 5). Ebenso untersuchten Scherer et al. (14) die Beziehung zwischen Metallallergie und Prothesenlockerung und erfragten bei 33,1% eine positive Allergieanamnese und von denen, die eine Metallallergie angaben waren 27% im Epikutantest positiv, dagegen Patienten mit unspezifischer bekannter Allergie zu 18,2%. Die häufigsten Reaktionen im Hauttest wurden bei Cobalt mit 42,9% und Nickelsulfat 38,1%, Kaliumdichromat 14,3% beobachtet. Gleichzeitig wird berichtet, dass die Sensibilisierungsrate bei 248 Ersteingriffen bei 4,2% und bei 102 Revisionen der Hüftimplantate bei 10,8% lag. Weitere Revisionsoperationen zeigten eine geringere Zunahme (3. Op – 12,5%) der positiven Patch-Testung. Zu beachten ist die Kontaktallergie auf Metall bei Patienten mit einem Ekzem, wobei nach Implantation ein lokales Ekzem zu beobachten ist (4). Bei akutem Auftreten von lokalisierten oder generalisierten Erythemata, Urticaria, Ekzeme oder in seltenen Fällen, Vaskulitiden (7) muss an eine Beziehung zum Implantat gedacht werden.

Kasuistiken

1. Patient: B. B. geb. 30.1. 39 (Abb. 1 – 3)

1. OP
   - wegen Dysplasiecoxarthrose nach Eigenblutspende im Okt. 96 Implantation einer Hüft-TEP li. (Zweymüller-Titan-Schaft zementfrei und Schraubpfanne mit Metasul Metall-Metall-Gleitpaarung), primäre Wundheilung, AHB, keine Vorsensibilisierung bekannt
   - 4 Wo. nach AHB spontane Wunddehiszenz (Tab. **1**)
2. – 5. OP
   - Revisionen mit Entfernung von Nahtmaterial insges. 4 × notwendig (chromierte Fäden)
   - Nickelsensibilisierung nachgewiesen
6. OP
   - Wechsel der Metasulgleitpaarung am 10. 3. 98 gegen Keramikkopf (Bionit) und Polyethylen (UHMWPE)-Inlay wegen anhaltender Hüftschmerzen li.
   - Prednisolongabe zwischenzeitlich war effektlos.
   - Erneute Wundheilungsstörung mit
7. OP
   - Wundrevision am 26. 3. 98.
8. OP
   - Erneute Schmerzen wegen Lockerung des Zweymüller-Schaftes, proximale Femurfraktur.
   - Wechsel in R + V-Prothese am 7. 8. 98
   - verzögerte Wundheilung.
9. OP
   - Entfernung der Verriegelungsschrauben Sept. 99
   - z. Z. keine Beschwerden.

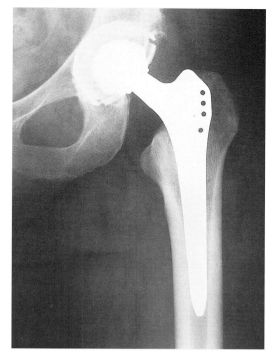

Abb. 1 1996

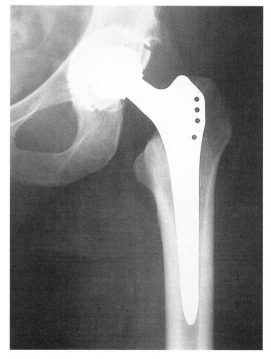

Abb. 2 1998

3.1 Hypersensitivity in THR: A Case Study

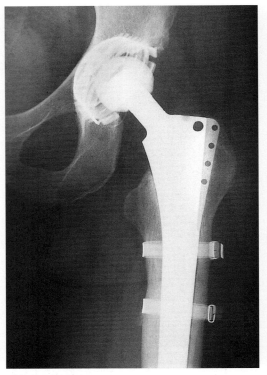

Abb. 3   1999

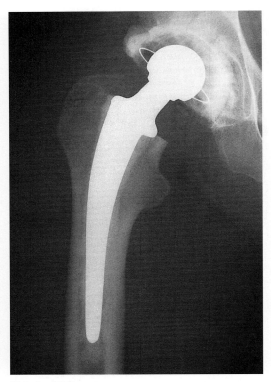

Abb. 4   1985

Tab. 1

Epikutantest: einfach positive Reaktion:	24	48	72 h
– Endoprothese Polyethylen	∅	∅	∅
– Endoprothese Metal	∅	∅	∅
– Titan	∅	∅	∅
– Endoprothese Keramik (Aluminiumhydroxyd)	∅	∅	∅
– Palacos	∅	∅	∅
– Nahtmaterial Catgut 2	∅	∅	∅
– Polyester 0	∅	∅	∅
– Sutupak	∅	∅	∅
– Dexon	∅	∅	∅
– Kaliumdichromat	∅	∅	∅
– Nickelsulfat	+	+	+
– Ti 6 A/7 NB	∅	∅	∅
– Ti A/4 C	∅	∅	∅
– S 30	∅	∅	∅
– Ti	∅	∅	∅
– CoCr	∅	∅	∅
– Berlosin	∅	∅	∅

2. Patient: A. R. geb. 25. 9. 25 (Abb. 4 – 6)

1. OP
   - Wegen Coxarthrose bds. mit Hüftkopfnekrose Implantation einer zementierten Protecast-Prothese (CrCoMo) mit Polyethylen-Pfanne zementiert re. 5/85.
   - 2 Tage postop. juckendes papulöses Exanthem am ganzen Körper, nach Gabe von Prednisolon + Antibiotika Rückgang der Hauterscheinungen,
   - verzögerte Wundheilung,
   - keine Vorsensibilisierung spez. bekannt, empfindlich auf bestimmte Obstsorten.
2. OP
   - anhaltende Trochanterschmerzen deshalb Trochanterrevision 1/87 re.,
   - weil Hauteffluresezenzen abgeheilt, jetzt Epikutan-Test (Tab. 2).
3. OP
   - Da Prothesen- und Pfannenlockerung Wechsel in Titanschaft mit Keramik-Kopf und erneut zementierte Polyethylenpfanne am 9.1.89.

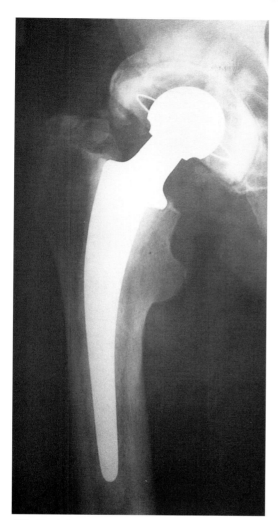

Abb. 5 1987

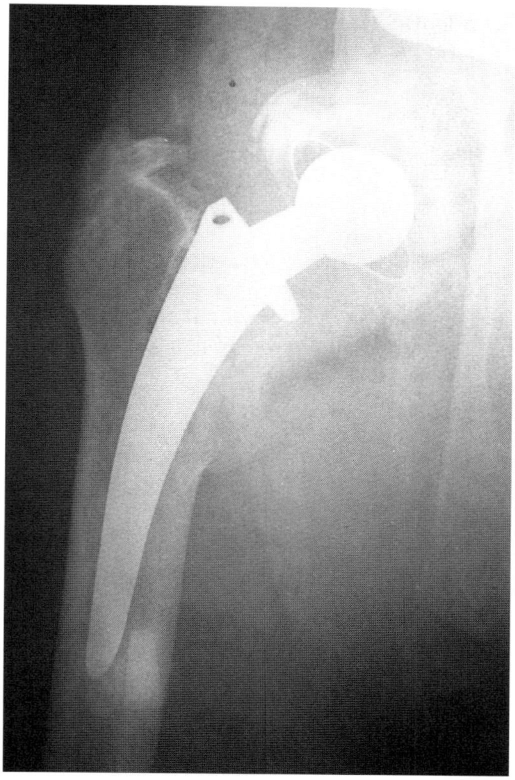

Abb. 6 1989

Tab. 2

Epikutantest: einfach positive Reaktion:	24	48	72 h
– Hüftpfanne	∅	∅	∅
– Keramikkopf	∅	∅	∅
– Prothesenschaft	∅	+	+
– Perlon	∅	+	+

3. Patient: L.L. geb. 12.6.32 (Abb. 7, 8)

1. OP
   - Wegen Achsfehlstellung des li. Knie 4/94 li. TKKO.
2. OP
   - progrediente schmerzhafte Gonarthrose, deshalb Implantation eines Foundation-Knee li. am 28.11.96,
   - am 3. Tag starke Schwellung und Rötung li. Knie mit distalem Oberschenkel und proximalem Unterschenkel mit allergischem Exanthem, Prednisolon-Gabe von 75 mg/die absteigend für ½ Jahr,
   - Sensibilisierung durch Osteosynthesematerial bei TKKO
3. OP
   - wegen Gonarthrose rechts am 20.2.98 Implantation eines Natural-Knee re.
   - am 2. Tag postop. Schwellung und Rötung, Behandlung mit Prednisolon von 50 mg/dies absteigend.

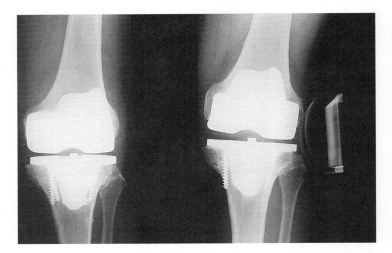

Abb. 7 1998

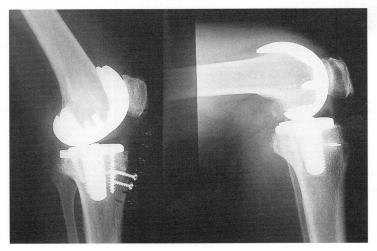

Abb. 8 1999

Diskussion

In einer Befragung unserer stationären Patienten gaben 18% Überempfindlichkeitsreaktionen der Haut auf Obst, Waschmittel usw. an. 4,6% konnten exakte Angaben über eine Nickel-Allergie und 1,5% über eine Chrom-Allergie ausführen. Diese liegen unter den getesteten Allergieraten von Scherer et al. (14). Es ist deshalb rückzuschließen, dass nach Durchführung eines generellen Epikutan-Testes für alle potentiellen Implantatträger eine Angleichung der Häufigkeitszahlen eintritt.

Seit Sept. 1995 implantieren wir die Metall-Metall-Hartpaarung Metasul durchschnittlich bei 42 Patienten jährlich. Obwohl die übrigen Implantatanteile bei der erstgenannten Patientin kein Nickel enthielten, bewirkte der Nickel/Chrom-Anteil in der Metasul-Gleitpaarung die Reaktionen, die als Nickelallergie gedeutet wurde. Sie wurde aber nicht objektiviert durch den Epikutantest. Folgende Nachweise bei Verdacht auf ein haematogenes allergisches Kontaktekzem durch eine Nickelallergie bei Totalendoprothesenimplantation haben sich bewährt:
- Epikutantest
- Nachweis von T-Lymphozyten im Blut, die nur auf Nickel sensible Antikörper aufweisen
- klonale Bestimmung spezifisch sensibilisierter T-Lymphozyten
- LTT = Lymphozytentransformationstest, mit Vorgabe einer spezifischen Sensibilisierung von T-Lymphozyten

Im Epikutantest der o. gen. Patientin konnte kein Anstieg der Reaktion festgestellt werden. Die stattgehabte Reaktion ist nicht beweisend, denn eine Sensibilisierung bei fehlender Verstärkung der cutanen Reaktion kann auch z.B. durch Trinkwasser, Mehl und viele andere Substanzen bedingt sein. Die Attribute einer Kontaktallergie auf das Implantat fehlen (4,7). Die röntgenologisch eingetretene Lockerung des Implantates ist ebenfalls nicht als Folge einer Reaktion auf die Bestandteile der Implantate zurückzuführen (15, 7,12).

Am Beispiel des Pat. A.R. nach Epikutantest vom Material des Prothesenschaftes und Nahtmaterial ist eine einfach positive Reaktion festgestellt, der verwendete Keramikkopf sowie die Polyethylenpfanne bewirkten keine cutane Reaktion. Die Lockerung des Schaftes aus CrCoMo ist entsprechend der Untersuchungen von Wilke et al. (17) auch eine Folge eines verminderten Zellwachstums an den Grenzflächen mit verminderter Produktion von extrazellulärer Matrix und führte zum berichteten Wechsel. Neben der Wirkung von Abriebpartikeln von Polyethylen und Metallegierungen bewirken letztere einen Anstieg der Cytokine, die ebenfalls Osteolysen induzieren (8) können. Eine zytotoxische Wirkung der oben genannten Materialien stört den Vorgang der Einheilung der Implantate (17). Die Folge einer allergischen Reaktion mit dadurch bedingter Lockerung des Schaftes der Prothese ist schon wegen der fehlenden Langhanszellen vor Ort nicht möglich. Mechanische Einflüsse bei Granulozytenwirkung periprothetisch sind die häufigsten Lockerungsursachen.

Eine Knochenreaktion wurde beim 3. beschriebenen Patienten nach Kniegelenksimplantation trotz heftiger lokaler Reaktion bis dato nicht konstatiert. Die frühzeitige Subpression durch hohe Gaben von Corticosteroiden haben eine normale Einheilung der Titanoberfläche im Knochen gesichert. Die starke synoviale Reaktion wurde den Gleitflächen des Kniegelenkes aus CrCo angelastet. Auf Grund des beschriebenen Krankheitsverlaufes muss diese Einschätzung jedoch entsprechend zurückhaltend interpretiert werden.

Literatur

1. Benson MKD, Goodwin PG, Brostoff J (1975) Metal sensibility in patients with joint replacement arthroplastics. BMJ 4, 374–375
2. Caciller F, De Giorgis P, Verdoia C, Parrini L, Lodi A, Croasti C (1992) Allergy to components of total hip arthroplasty before and after surgery. Ital. J. Orthop. Traumatol. 18, 407–410
3. Carlsson AS, Magnusson B, Möller H (1980) Metal sensitivity in patients with metal-to-plastic total hip arthroplastic. Acta Orthop. Scand. 51, 57–62
4. Carlsson A, Moeller H (1989) Implantation of orthopedic devica in patients with metal allergy. Acta Derm. Venerol. (Stockholm) 69, 62–66
5. Deutman R, Mulder TJ, Brian R, Nater JP (1977) Metal sensitivity before und after total hip arthroplasty. J. Bone Joint Surg. Am. 59, 862–865
6. Fink U (1997) Sicherheitsaspekte bei der Beschichtung von Titangleitkomponenten. Orthopäde 26, 160–165
7. Gawrodger DJ (1993) Nickel sensitivity and the Implantation of orthopedic prosthesis. Contact Dermatitis 28, 257–259

8. Haynes D, Rogers SD, Hay S, Pearcy MJ, Howie DW (1993) The differences in toxity and release of boneresorbing mediafors induced by titanium and cobalt-chromium-Alloy wear particles. J. Bone Joint Surg. A 75-A 825–834
9. Jacobs JJ, Skipor AK, Doorn PF, Cambell P, Schmalzried TP, Black J, Amstutz HC (1996) Cobalt and Chronium concentrations in patients with metal on metal total hip replacements. Clin. Orthop. Relat. Res. 329, 256–263
10. Merrit K, Brown SA (1996) Distribution of Cobalt Chronium wear and corrosion products and biologic reactions. Clin. Orthop. Relat. Res. 329, 233–243
11. Merrit K, Brown SA (1984) Effect of valence of chromium on biogical responses In: Ducheyne P, Van der Perre G, Aubert AE (eds.) Biomaterials and biomechanics. Elsevier, Amsterdam
12. Milavec C, Puretic V, Orlic D, Marusic A (1998) Sensitivity to metals in 40 patients with failed hip endoprosthesis. Arch Orthop. Trauma Surg. 117, 383–386
13. Plitz W, Huber J, Refior HJ (1997) Experimentelle Untersuchungen an Metall-Metall-Gleitpaarungen und ihre Wertigkeit hinsichtlich eines zu erwartenden In-vivo-Verhaltens. Orthopäde 26, 135–141
14. Scherer MA, Cheung-Chi-Wing J, Rothe M, Lechner F (1990) Metallallergie und Prothesenlockerung – Gibt es Zusammenhänge? In: Die gelockerte Hüftprothese. Hrsg. Ascherl R, Schattauer, Stuttgart, New York, 198–209
15. Török L, Greczy I, Ocsai H, Czako J (1995) Investigation into the development of allergy to metal in recipients of implanted hip prosthesis a prospective study. Eur. Dermatol. 5, 294–295
16. Walter A (1997) Die Keramik-Keramik-Paarung. Orthopäde 26, 110–116
17. Wilke A, Hirschheydt SV, Orth J, Kienapfel H, Griss P, Franke RP (1995) Die humane Knochenmarkszellkultur – eine sensitive Methode zur Beurteilung der Biokompartibilität von Materialien, die in der Orthopädie verwendet werden. Z. Orthop. 133, 159–165
18. Wilkinson DS, Wilkinson JD (1979) Comparison of patch test results in two adjacent areas of England. Acta Dermato. Vener. 59, 189–191
19. Zichner L, Lindenfeld T (1997) In-vivo-Verschleiß der Gleitpaarungen Keramik-Polyethylen gegen Metall-Polyethylen. Orthopäde 26, 129–134

3.2 Clinical Relevance of Allergological Tests in Total Joint Replacement

M. Schramm, R. P. Pitto

Abstract

Adverse hypersensitive reactions due to biomaterial allergy are a concern for orthopaedic surgeons. In total joint replacement allergic mechanisms are discussed as possible reason for eczematous reactions, early aseptic loosening and postoperative complications, such as wound healing disturbances or delayed bone healing. The recommendation that patients with cutaneous hypersensitivity having a total joint replacement should receive a prosthesis made of anallergic biomaterial is common. Nevertheless, little is known about the clinical relevance of positive allergological tests and cutaneuos reactions in orthopaedics. To investigate this special topic we performed a systematic review of the current literature. The Medline bibliographic database was reviewed from 1974 to 1999 to identify all the relevant literature. The analysis included a total of 1058 patients in 16 peer-reviewed papers. There were 3 controlled studies, 14 prospective and 4 retrospective trials. We found 12 review papers, 4 experimental studies and 2 case reports.

Specificity and sensibility of usual epicutaneous patch-tests seems to be low due to the different reactive potential of skin and bone, and no correlation could be found between positive skin testing and any postoperative complications. There is no relevant routine test to diagnose allergic reaction to biomaterials in the blood. Nowadays, the use of titanium alloy in patients who have been sensitized to nickel, chromium, and cobalt is generally advocated.

For revision arthroplasty in cases of aseptic loosening of cemented prostheses fixation using cementless technique should be preferred. Prevention of adverse allergic reactions can be achieved by reducing the production of biomaterial debris due to wear, fretting and corrosion. Thus, biomaterials with adequate tribological behaviour and stable fixation of the prosthesis components are the best prophylactic measure to manage hypersensitivity in total joint replacement.

Knowledge regarding hypersensitivity in total joint replacement is based on little evident data. Controlled clinical trials are required in order to provide additional informations on the efficacy of treatment outcome.

Introduction

Adverse reactions due to biomaterial allergy are a concern for orthopaedic surgeons ever since Laugier and Foussereau [15] described the first case of dermatitis following osteosynthesis with a plate in 1964. Dermatitis following orthopaedic operations has been described in 54 cases (Fig. 1) [21]. In total joint replacement allergic mechanisms are also discussed as possible reason for cases of early aseptic loosening without mechanical explanation. The pathogenesis of this event is not yet clear. Does allergy cause loosening or does loosening cause allergy? Distinction of metal related allergy or cell toxicity remains difficult.

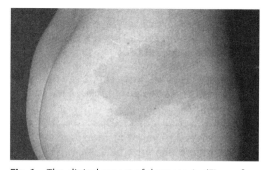

Fig. 1 The clinical aspect of dermatosis. (Figure from EG Jung (1989) Dematologie, Hippokrates Verlag, Stuttgart, 55).

Which type of allergic reactions are responsible? What are appropriate tests?

This paper represents a review of the current literature to collect relevant informations concerning biomaterial allergy in orthopaedic surgery. We try to deduct some guidelines for the proper management of total joint replacement patients.

Material and Method

We have performed a systematic review of the current literature. The Medline bibliographic database (Pubmed®) was reviewed from 1974 to 1999 to identify all the relevant literature. The analysis included a total of 1058 patients in 16 peer-reviewed papers. There were 3 controlled studies, 14 prospective and 4 retrospective trials. We found 12 review papers, 4 experimental studies and 2 case reports.

Physiopathology and Diagnosis

In most of the patients with a stated allergy, the diagnosis was verified by epicutaneous patch tests or intracutaneous scratch tests performed on the patient's back (Fig. 2). Standard batteries of metals and other biomaterials tested for allergic reactions include chromium, nickel, cobalt and titanium. According to case reports or studies on small numbers of patients allergy reactions are as well possible to non-metalic components of the prosthesis. Cutaneous tests should therefore include polyethylene and some components of bone cement, especially mono- and polymers of methylmethacrylate [19] and N,N-dimethyl-paratoluidine (DMT), an accelerator substance of bone cement [12]. Some authors found considerable sensitivity to vanadium, which is used in some alloys of hip prostheses [3]. The reactive potential of tissues decreases from skin to mucous membranes and subcutaneous tissue. Due to the low reactive potential of bone, positive patch-test results do not necessarily have a clinical relevance for the orthopaedic surgeon [10].

Insertion of small devices made of the same material as the designated prosthesis into subcutaneous tissue generates unspecific granulomatous reactions and can not be clinically distinguished from hypersensitivity. In dentistry reaction to materials are tested by long-term exposition to mucous tissue in the mouth. Both methods do not give relevant informations concerning the prognosis of bone reaction to orthopaedic implants [10].

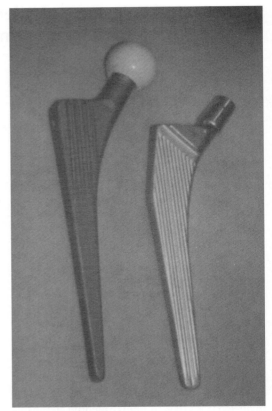

Fig. 2 Schematic presentation of epicutaneous patch testing to evaluate hypersensitivity to hip prostheses made of different alloys.

There are no routine blood tests that specifically prove the presence of allergic reactions. In immunohistochemical studies the labelling of macrophages, T-lymphocytes and B-lymphocytes by monoclonal antibodies may identify the distribution and frequency of these cells. This can indicate sensitisation [14]. Blood test related changes consist of lymphopenia with reduced subpopulations of CD4 and CD8 and decreased in-vitro cytotoxic activity. These changes can be interpreted as cell mediated hypersensitivity or as well as toxic effect of ions released from the implant [11]. Carando et al. proposed a specific lymphocytic transformation tests in 1985, but could not gain broad acceptance due to the complexity of the method [4].

The ionic forms of Ni, Co and Cr are known to cause contact eczema [17]. Possible reactions attributable to allergy range from aseptic loosening, disturbance of wound healing to certain forms of dermatitis. Skin reactions include eczematous reactions of dermatitis (44%), bullous dermatosis (11%), cellulitis (13%) [9], sterile abscesses around the implant [21] and various less frequent lesions. Infection is not generated by metal allergy, but septic loosening results via increased corrosion in a higher rate of sensitisation to metals [13]. The definite classification of skin lesions as orthopaedic dermatosis can be made only after implant removal. All of the criteria depicted in Table **1** must be fulfilled.

Table 1 Criteria for diagnosis of orthopaedic dermatosis [21]

Orthopaedic dermatosis
1. Definitive form of dermatosis following insertion of an implant
2. No other possible etiology despite additional research
3. Chronic dermatosis
4. Healing of dermatosis within 2 months after implant removal
5. Corrosion of removed implant (microscopy, spectrophotometry, positive spot test, wear products)

Immune response in form of allergy usually needs certain preconditions. Corrosion leads to particulate debris of prosthesis material, which migrates into the membranes of the surrounding tissue [21]. The metal ions can act as haptens, link to dermal proteins and induce immunization. That provokes mainly delayed hypersensitivity (type IV). Cr- and Ni-ions have a cytotoxic effect on fibroblasts and lymphocytes, they cause lymphoblastic transformation. Ni- and Co-ions trigger the degranulation of mast- and basophil cells and impair the function of macrophages. Immediate hypersensitivity (type I) can be observed and lead to urticaria. Vasculitis can be secondary to immunecomplex deposit (type III) or to the liberation of lymphokines (type IV) [21].

For the definitive diagnosis of delayed allergic reaction (type IV) the metal incriminated by allergologic tests, the metal found in the tissue surrounding the implant, and the material of the implant must be concordant A type I reaction can also be characterized by a positive basophil degranulation test [21].

The Relevance of Patch Testing

Prospective studies on epicutaneous patch tests in patients receiving an arthroplasty were performed since 1976 [2, 20]. None of those could state a correlation between skin hypersensitivity and loosening of components or local side effects like dermatitis following surgery. A recent prospective study concerning the significance of contact sensitization caused by metal implants was presented in 1998 by Duchna et al. [8]. They have performed patch tests preoperatively and 1 year after surgery in 100 patients matched into 3 groups: patients receiving a) titanium hip implants or b) stainless steel implants (nickel-alloys) and c) patients who had surgery without any implants. Three of these 100 patients presented a nickel-allergy before surgery. Of them, 2 had received nickel-alloy containing implants while one was treated using a titanium implant. None developed a postoperative complication related to the allergy. Onset of allergy to nickel or chromium was observed in 3 other patients after operation. Two of them had received a titanium implant and both showed postoperative complications. A possible source of the allergy was wear of metal-containing jewelry. The other patient developed a specific allergy to the same metal as his endoprosthesis was made, but no postoperative complication occurred. In conclusion, no correlation of specific metal-allergy and postoperative complications was found.

In 1989 Carlsson and Moller [5] followed 18 patients with preoperatively patch-test-verified allergy against alloys of the prostheses used over a mean of 6.3 years. None had suffered any dermatologic or orthopaedic complication.

Granchi et al. evaluated results of epicutaneous patch testing in 16 patients with aseptic loosening of hip arthroplasty. Only one patch test was postive, again there was no correlation [11].

Allergy and Aseptic Loosening of Implants

Periprosthetic osteolysis caused by wear debris released from the bearing surface of polyethylene components (Fig. 3) is one of the major issues in total hip and knee arthroplasty [1]. Data on the role of hypersensitivity for aseptic loosening of the implant are controversial. Hip prostheses with a metal-metal bearing used in the 1960s induced sensitivity to metals in 28–46% of cases [2,18,20]. Modern metal-polyethylene (PE) bearings induce allergy according to skin tests in 3–10% [6,7]. In 1998 a study on 40 patients with failed hip arthroplasty due to aseptic loosening was presented [18]. The authors compared 9 patients with positive patch tests for Cr, Co, Ni or rust to 31 patients with no positive cutaneous allergy tests. There was no significant difference between the two groups in age, sex, reasons and number of revisions, implant function, type of prosthesis or bearing surface (metal-metal, metal-PE), circulating immunecomplexes and histologic findings in the surrounding tissue. Chronic granulomatous non specific inflammation was the mean finding. They concluded that hypersensitivity to metals does not play a significant role in the loosening of the endoprosthesis. Thus, the instability of the prosthesis generates an increased amount of wear debris and leads to hypersensitivity reactions [17,18].

Lewin et al. used Guinea pigs sensitized to nickel, cobalt, or chromium to study if impaired fixation occurres as a result of metal allergy. Screws were inserted in the tibiae, and the mechanical strength of the fixation to the bone was evaluated after 4 months. To see if changes in bone density occurred in the proximal tibia as a result of allergy, the amount of ash was determined. Although the animals maintained their contact sensitivity throughout the experimental period, there were no differences between allergic and control animals for any of the parameters studied. The experiment indicates that contact allergy may be unimportant for the fate of orthopedic implants [16].

Besides metal hypersensitivity, allergic tissue reactions are also possible to polyethylene or some components of bone cement [17]. Haddad et al. verified the role of N,N-dimethyl-paratoluidine (DMT), an accelerator substance of bone cement as an indicator for rapid aseptic loosening [12]. Seven of 70 patients in his controlled study were patch test positive to DMT, all presented aseptic loosening of the cemented component of the arthroplasty. Three of the patients with DMT hypersensitivity showed again aseptic loosening after revision arthroplasty performed using cement. They considered DMT hypersensitivity a primary phenomen, because it was not found in any of the patients of the control group with septic loosening.

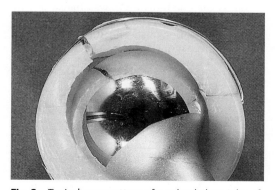

Fig. 3 Typical wear pattern of a polyethylene inlay after retrieval. Production of polyethylene debris represents one of the major causes of aseptic loosening in total joint replacement.

The Safety of Titanium Implants

Titanium implants are usually considered a safe option for patients with suspected allergy to Ni, Cr or Co [21]. Nevertheless, Lalor et al. postulated that sensitivity to titanium might lead to implant failure [14]. This is the only report regarding allergic reactions of bone to titanium-alloy implants. They investigated 5 cases with loosened titanium implants using mouse anti-human monoclonal antibodies. Additionally electron microscopy was performed. Within the membranes surrounding the removed implant they found abundant macrophages and T-lymphocytes response, but no B-Lymphocytes or plasma cells, and only few granulocytes. This indicates cell mediated (type IV) hypersensitivity reactions. None of the 5 patients had positive patch tests to any titanium salts, which is a contradiction to the demonstrated type IV reaction. Blackened mem-

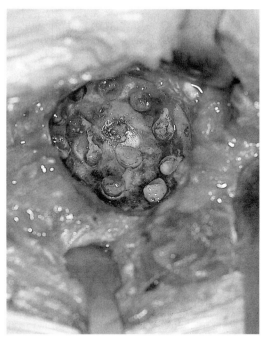

Fig. 4 Periarticular granulomatous membranes containing titanium debris in a patient with aseptic loosening of a cementless acetabular component.

branes caused by titanium wear debris are well known in revision surgery (Fig. **4**). From the histological point of view, this finding seems to be not related to allergic but to granulomatous reactions.

Conclusions

Due to the different reactive potential of skin and bone the specificity and sensibility of current patch-tests are insufficient. None of the studies reviewed could clearly demonstrate a significant correlation between positive patch- or prick testing to metals and postoperative complications after implantation of a total hip replacement [2, 5, 8, 11, 20].

There is no relevant routine blood test to diagnose allergic reaction to metals. Even when using antibody-related tests for cells of the immune systeme, the definitive differentiation of allergy and cell toxicity remains difficult [4, 11, 14].

The rare condition of orthopaedic dermatosis can be proved only after removal of the implant [9, 21].

Allergic reactions to titanium are uncommon. Thus, the use of titanium alloy for implants in patients who have been sensitized to nickel, chromium, and cobalt is advocated [14, 21].

Due to possible hypersensitivity reactions to certain components of bone cement, such as DMT, revision arthroplasty following aseptic loosening of cemented implants should be performed using cementless technique [12].

It is generally recognized, that the most important mean to prevent allergy mediated dermatosis is to reduce production of metalic particles due to wear, fretting and corrosion [1, 9, 17]. Primary stable implants with carefully selected bearing couples, that produce as little debris as possible are the best preventive measure for any allergic reaction in arthroplasty.

In conclusion, the state of the art concerning hypersensitivity in total joint replacement is based on little evident data. Controlled clinical trials are required, in order to provide additional informations regarding outcome of patients with pre-existent hypersensitivity to biomaterials used in total joint replacement surgery.

References

1 Amstutz HC, Grigoris P (1996) Metal on metal bearings in hip arthroplasty. Clin Orthop Suppl. 329: 11 – 34
2 Brown GC, Lockshin MD, Salvati EA, Bullough PG (1977) Sensitivity to metal as possible cause of sterile loosening after cobalt-chromium total hip-replacement arthroplasty. J Bone Joint Surg 59 A: 164 – 168
3 Cancilleri F, De Giorgis P, Verdoia C, Parrini L, Lodi A, Crosti C (1992) Allergy to components of total hip arthroplasty before and after surgery. Ital J Orthop Traumatol 18: 407 – 10
4 Carando S, Cannas M, Rossi P, Portigliatti-Barbos M (1985) The lymphocytic transformation test (L. T. T.) in the evaluation of intolerance in prosthetic implants. Ital J Orthop Traumatol 11: 475 – 481
5 Carlsson A, Moller H (1989) Implantation of orthopaedic devices in patients with metal allergy. Acta Derm Vernereol 69: 62 – 66
6 Carlsson AS, Magnusson B, Moller H (1980) Metal sensitivity in patients with metal-to-plastic total hip arthroplasties. Acta Orthop Scand 51: 57 – 62

7. Deutmann R, Mulder TJ, Brian R, Nater JP (1977) Metal sensitivity before and after total hip arthroplasty. J Bone Joint Surg 59 A: 862–865
8. Duchna HW, Nowack U, Merget R, Muhr G, Schuktze-Werninghaus G (1998) Prospective study of the significance of contact sensitization caused by metal implants. Zentralblatt Chirurgie 123: 1271–76
9. Dujardin F, Février V, Lecorvaisier C, Joly P (1995) Dermatoses d'intolerance aux implants métalliques en chirurgie orthopédique. Revue de Chirurgie Orthopédique 81: 473–484
10. Fartasch M (2000) personal communication
11. Granchi D, Ciapetti G, Stea S, Cavedagna D, Bettini N, Bianco T, Fontanesi G, Pizzoferrato A (1995) Evaluation of several immunological parameters in patients with aseptic loosening of hip arthroplasty. Chir Organi Mov 80: 399–408
12. Haddad FS, Cobb AG, Bentley G, Levell NJ, Dowd PM (1996) Hypersensitivity in aseptic loosening of total hip replacements. The role of constituents of bone cement. J Bone Joint Surg 78 B: 546–549
13. Hierholzer S, Hierholzer G (1982) Allergy to metal following osteosynthesis. Unfallchirurgie 8: 347–352
14. Lalor PA, Revell PA, Gray AB, Wright S, Railton GT, Freeman MA (1991) Sensitivity to titanium. A cause of implant failure? J Bone Joint Surg 73 B: 25–28
15. Laugier P, Foussereau J, Bulte C (1964) L'allergie au nickel du matériel d'osteosynthèse. Soc Dermatol Syph 71: 691–694 (citation according to 9)
16. Lewin J, Lindgren JU, Wahlberg JE (1987) Apparent absence of local response to bone screws in guinea pigs with contact sensitivity. J Orthop Res 5: 604–608
17. Merritt K, Brown SA (1996) Distribution of cobalt chromium wear and corrosion products and biologic reactions. Clin Orthop 329 Suppl: 233–243
18. Milavec-Puretic V, Orlic D, Marusic A (1998) Sensitivity to metals in 40 patients with failed hip endoprosthesis. Arch Orthop Trauma Surg 117: 383–386
19. Monteny E, Oleffe J, Donkerwolke M (1978) Methylmethacrylate hypersensitivity in a patient with cemented endoprosthesis. A case report. Acta Orthop Scan 49: 554–556
20. Nater JP, Brain RG, Deutman R, Mulder TJ (1976) The development of metal hypersensitivity in patients with metal-to-plastic hip arthroplasties. Contact Dermatosis 2: 259–261
21. Rostocker G, Robin J, Binet O, Blamoutier J, Paupe J, Lessana-Leibowitch M, Bedouelle J, Sonneck JM, Garrel JB, Millet P (1987) Dermatosis due to Orthopaedic Implants – A review of the literature and report of three cases. J Bone Joint Surg 69 A: 1408–1412

3.3 Whole-Blood Cobalt and Chromium Levels in Patients Managed with Total Hip Replacements Involving Different Metal-on-Metal Combinations

C. Lhotka, J. Steffan, K. Zhuber, T. Szekeres, K. Zweymüller

Abstract

Metal-on-metal combinations in total hip prostheses produce a small amount of wear. This is why we followed up the whole-blood levels of cobalt and chromium, in 219 patients (mean age: 54 years), over a period of 38 months post-arthroplasty, using atomic absorption spectrometry. Of the patients in the study, 106 had been given an implant made by Manufacturer No. 1, while 97 had been given an implant made by Manufacturer No. 2. Age- and gender-matched subjects without hip replacements and free of any other major orthopaedic hardware were used as a control group. Compared with the controls, all the patients had significantly higher cobalt and chromium levels. Thus, cobalt and chromium wear debris was demonstrated in the blood following hip replacement with either device. As a result, we recommend that patients managed with a metal-on-metal combination THR be monitored at regular intervals with clinical and radiological examinations, to detect local or systemic reactions early on.

Introduction

One of the requirements to be met by total hip replacements is that they should produce little wear. Implant longevity is predicated upon a low wear rate of the femoral head and the cup (Doorn [1], Amstutz [2]; Streicher [3]; Bergmann [4]; Plitz [5], Thomsen [6], Müller [7]). The cobalt and chromium wear debris produced by metal-on-metal combinations differs from polyethylene wear debris in that it is carried from the production site into the bloodstream. (Merritt [8], Baslé [9]). This is why cobalt and chromium levels in the blood will allow the wear rate of the bearing surfaces to be inferred. Our study was performed to determine whether there is time-dependent metal wear; and if so, what the wear rate is. We also wanted to see whether there is a "bedding-in" phase, and whether there are differences between devices involving metal-on-metal combinations made by different manufacturers. It was decided to compare metal-on-metal combinations made by two different manufacturers, and to measure the ion levels in the blood at different times post-arthroplasty.

Material and Methods

Patients

All the patients in the study were managed with a cementless titanium stem of rectangular cross-section, and a threaded titanium cup. The devices used were made by the two most important manufacturers in Europe. One hundred and six patients had been given a total hip replacement made by Manufacturer No. 1; 97 patients had been given a total hip replacement made by Manufacturer No. 2. Of the patients who had been managed with a device by Manufacturer No. 1, 60 were female, and 46 were male; the mean age was 53.5 years, and the mean body weight 63,8 kg. Of the patients who had been managed with a device by Manufacturer No. 2, 60 were female, and 37 were male; the mean age was 56 years, and the mean body weight 74.5 kg. The control group comprised 31 healthy subjects, of whom 24 were female, and seven were male; the mean age was 52 years, and the mean body weight 68.5 kg. The THR patients and the healthy controls were consented, following which blood samples were taken and assayed for whole-blood levels of cobalt and chromium. The patients were divided into four groups with different sampling times: in Group I, the assay was performed immediately post-arthroplasty; in Group II, at 3–6 months; in Group III, at 12–15 months; and in Group IV, at 35–38 months post-arthroplasty.

Method

The assays were performed using freeze-dried ashed whole blood. Each sample was subjected to three measurements with GFAAS (graphite tube atom absorption spectrometry) (Perkin Elmar 4100). GFAAS was chosen because of its very wide dynamic range, and because of its ability to determine main and ancillary elements and to demonstrate traces and ultra-traces.

Results

Cobalt

The healthy control group (n = 31) had a mean cobalt level of 0.7 ng/g. Of the 106 patients who had been managed with a device made by Manufacturer No. 1, the 24 patients in Group I (immediate post-arthroplasty assay) had a mean cobalt level (± S.D.) of 3.22 (± 2.00) ng/g. Group II (n = 27), assayed at 3–6 months, had a mean level of 10.87 (± 3.14) ng/g. Group III (n = 27), assayed at 12–15 months, had a mean level of 23.34 (± 6.94) ng/g. Group IV (n = 28), assayed at 35–38 months, had a mean level of 36.54 (± 10.15) ng/g (Fig. 1).

Of the 97 patients who had been managed with a device made by Manufacturer No. 2, the 24 patients in Group I (immediate post-arthroplasty assay) had a mean cobalt level (± S.D.) of 8.13 (± 4.93) ng/g. Group II (n = 24), assayed at 3–6 months, had a mean level of 14.04 (± 5.12) ng/g. Group III (n = 25), assayed at 12–15 months, had a mean level of 34.16 (± 16.34) ng/g. Group IV (n = 24), assayed at 35–38 months, had a mean level of 17.48 (± 7.33) ng/g (Fig. 2).

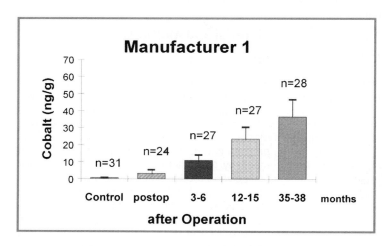

Fig. 1

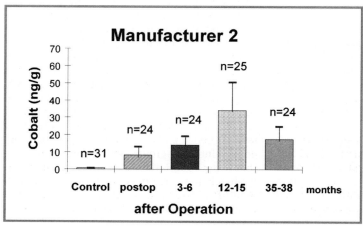

Fig. 2

Chromium

The pattern of chromium levels was similar to that observed with regard to cobalt.

The healthy controls had a mean chromium level of 0.21 ng/g.

Of the patients managed with a device made by Manufacturer No. 1, the 24 in Group I (immediate post-arthroplasty assay) had a mean chromium level (± S.D.) of 7.8 (± 2.91) ng/g. Group II (n = 27), assayed at 3–6 months, had a mean level of 16.8 (± 5.89) ng/g. Group III (n = 27), assayed at 12–15 months, had a mean level of 34.7 (± 7.84) ng/g. Group IV (n = 28), assayed at 35–38 months, had a mean level of 48.0 (± 14.07) ng/g (Fig. **3**).

Of the 97 patients who had been managed with a device made by Manufacturer No. 2, the 24 patients in Group I (immediate post-arthroplasty assay) had a mean chromium level (± S.D.) of 14.26 (± 6.61) ng/g. Group II (n = 24), assayed at 3–6 months, had a mean level of 21.63 (± 10.28) ng/g. Group III (n = 25), assayed at 12–15 months, had a mean level of 29.44 (± 13.67) ng/g. Group IV (n = 24), assayed at 35–38 months, had a mean level of 21.06 (± 8.98) ng/g (Fig. **4**).

Discussion

Metal-on-metal bearing combinations are popular in total hip replacement, because of their longevity and low wear rate. The alloys used initially had unduly high manufacturing tolerances, which made the implants (McKee [10]) less than optimal. For the past ten years or so, Manufacturer No. 1 has been using CoCr alloys with block carbides for his bearing surfaces, while Manufac-

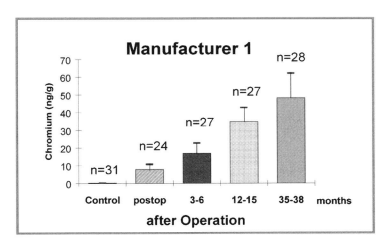

Fig. 3

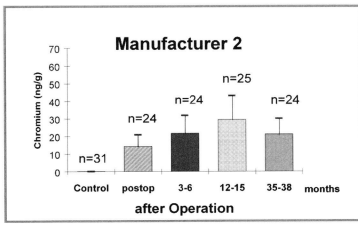

Fig. 4

turer No. 2 has, for the past five years, been using vacuum-melted CoCr alloys. Of the two metal-on-metal patterns in our study, some 100,000 have been implanted since 1988.

We studied the cobalt and chromium whole-blood levels in THR patients over a period of 38 months. This was done in order to see whether contemporary alloys will also produce measurable wear debris levels in the blood. We also wanted to see whether there was a difference in the wear behavior of implants made by the two different manufacturers. The wear observed during the follow-up period was in the nanogram range; however, at all times, the THR patients had significantly higher levels than did the controls.

Our results confirm the findings of Crawford [11], Brodner [12], Jacobs [13] and Lugowski [14], who, in serum studies conducted in smaller patient populations, observed significantly higher cobalt and chromium levels after total hip replacement involving metal-on-metal bearing combinations. In terms of the EKA values (exposure equivalents for cancerogenic substances) defined by the German group of investigators, some of the patients had cobalt levels in excess of what would be tolerated in industrial medicine (27.88 ng/g = 5 µg/L). It should, however, be borne in mind that the EKA values relate to respiratory exposure, and cannot, therefore, be readily translated to levels built up by direct ingress of the substances into the bloodstream. Apart from the possible cancerogenic effect of metal ions, as described by Gillespie [15], Lintner [16], Hicks [17] and Haynes [18], there is concern about possible local adverse effects. The adjacent tissue may mount an osteolytic response to metal wear debris, with local inflammatory, toxic and/or allergic reactions (Doorn [19], Agins [20], Buchert [21], Chan [22], Willert [23]). These reactions, in turn, would cause implant loosening. Although the cause-and-effect relationship between metal wear debris and systemic or local complications has not, to date, been established beyond doubt, metal wear debris must be suspected of inducing complications. This is why implants should be designed and manufactured in such a way as to produce minimal wear, and why patients who have been managed with THRs involving metal-on-metal bearing combinations should be monitored, at regular intervals, with clinical and radiological examinations.

References

1 Doorn, P. F., Campbell, P. A., Amstutz H. C.: Metal versus polyethylene wear particles in total hip replacements. A Review. Clin. Orthop. 329 S, 206–216, August 1996
2 Amstutz, H. C., Grigoris, P.: Metal on metal bearings in hip arthroplasty. Clin. Orthop. 329 S, 11–34, August 1996
3 Streicher, R. M., Schön, R., Semlitsch, M. F.: Untersuchung des tribologischen Verhaltens von Metall/Metall-Kombinationen für künstliche Hüftgelenke. Biomed. Technik, Band 35, Heft 5, 107–111, 1990
4 Bergmann, G., Graichen, F., Rohlmann, A.: Hip joint loading during walking and running measured in two patients. J. Biocmechanics, Vol. 26, No. 8, 969–990, 1993
5 Plitz, W., Huber, J., Refior, H. J.: Experimentelle Untersuchungen an Metall-Metall-Gleitpaarungen und ihre Wertigkeit hinsichtlich eines zu erwartenden In-vivo-Verhaltens. Orthopäde 26, 135–141, 1997
6 Thomsen, M., v. Strachwitz, B., Mau, H., Cotta, H.: Werkstoffübersicht in der Hüftendoprothetik. Z. Orthop. 133, 1–6, F. Enke Verlag Stuttgart 1995
7 Müller, M. E.: The benefits of metal-on-metal total hip replacements. Clin. Orthop. 311, 54–59, February 1995
8 Merritt, K., Brown, S. A.: Distribution of cobalt chromium wear and corrosion products and biologic reactions. Clin. Orthop. 329 S, 233–243, August 1996
9 Baslé, M. F., Bertrand, G., Guyetant, S., Chappard, D., Lesourd, M.: Migration of metal and polyethylene particles from articular prostheses may generate lymphadenopathy with histiocytosis. J. Biomedical Materials Research, Vol. 30, 157–164, 1996
10 McKee, G. K.: Total hip replacement – past, present and future. Biomaterials Vol. 3, 130–135, 1982
11 Crawford, R., Bonomo, T., Psychoyios, V., Delves, T., McLardy-Smith, P., Murray, D.: The serum level of cobalt chromium in a dynamic total hip replacement system. Nuffield Orthopaedic Centre, Headington, Oxford OX3 7 LD, England, at 8th Annual Meeting, European Orthopaedic Research Society, May 7–10, Amsterdam 1998
12 Brodner, W., Bitzan, P., Meisinger, V., Kaider, A., Gottsauner-Wolf F., Kotz, R.: Elevated serum cobalt with metal-on-metal articulating surfaces. Reprinted from: J. Bone Joint Surg. Vol. 79B, No. 2, 316–321, March 1997

13 Jacobs, J. J., Skipor, A. K., Black, J., Urban, R. M., Galante, J. O.: Release and excretion of metal in patients who have a total hip-replacement component made of titanium-base alloy. J. Bone Joint Surg. Vol. 73-A, No. 10, 1475–1485, December 1992
14 Lugowski, S. J., Smith, D. C., McHugh, A. D., Van Loon J. C.: Release of metal ions from dental implant materials in vivo: Determination of Al, Co, Cr, Mo, Ni, V, and Ti in organ tissue. J. Biomedical Materials Research, Vol. 25, 1443–1458, 1991
15 Gillespie, W. J., Henry, D. L., O'Connell, D., Kendrick, S., Juszczak, E., McInneny, K., Derby, L.: Development of Hematopoietic cancers after implantation of total joint replacement. Clin. Orthop. 329 S, 290–296, August 1996
16 Linter, F., Huber, M., Böhm, G., Attems, J., Lhotka, G.: Wertigkeit der Reaktionen des menschlichen Organismus auf freigesetzte Partikel im Rahmen der Endoprothesenimplantation. In: Zweymüller, K. (Hrsg.): Die Metall-Metall-Paarung Sikomet. Band 2., Verlag Hans Huber, 1999
17 Hicks, D. G., Judkins, A. R., Sickel, J. Z., Rosier, R. N., Puzas, J. E., O'Keefe R. J.: Granular histiocytosis of pelvic lymph nodes following total hip arthroplasty. J. Bone Joint Surg. Vol 78A, No. 4, 482–495, April 1996
18 Haynes, D. R., Rogers, S. D., Hay, S., Pearcy, M. J., Howie, D. W.: The differences in toxicity and release of bone-resorbing mediators induced by titanium and cobalt-chromium-alloy wear particles. J. Bone Joint Surg. Vol 75-A, No. 6, 825–833, June 1993
19 Doorn, P. F., Mirra, J. M., Campbell, P. A., Amstutz H. C.: Tissue reaction to metal on metal total hip prostheses. Clin. Orthop. 329 S, 187–205, August 1996
20 Agins, H. J., Alcock, N. W., Bansal, M., Salvati E. A., Wilson, P. D., Pellicci, P. M., Bullough, P. G.: Metallic wear in failed titanium-alloy total hip replacements. J. Bone Joint Surg. Vol 70-A, No. 3, 347–355, March 1988
21 Buchert, P. K., Vaughn, B. K., Mallory, T. H., Engh, C. A., Bobyn, J. D.: Excessive metal release due to loosening and fretting of sintered particles on porous-coated hip prostheses. J. Bone Joint Surg. Vol 68-A, No. 4, 606–609, April 1986
22 Chan, F. W., Bobyn, J. D., Medley, J. B., Krygier, J. J., Yue, St., Tanzer, M.: Engineering issues and wear performance of metal on metal hip implants. Clin. Orthop. 333, 96–107, 1996
23 Willert, H. G., Semlitsch, M.: Tissue reactions to plastic and metallic wear products of joint endoprostheses. Clin. Orthop. 333, 4–14, December, 1996

3.4 Biological Effects of Implanted Metallic Devices

J. Black, J. J. Jacobs

Introduction

Metallic alloys have been used for surgical implants for over a century. Despite the high chemical activity of fully reduced elements, as found in such implants, this practice has arisen due to the high strength and formability of metals. Through clinical experience and more recent laboratory and animal experimentation, device designers now have a variety of metallic materials suitable for acute and chronic implantation in repair and replacement of the musculoskeletal system.

The choice of metals for chronic implant applications is essentially made among three alloy systems: stainless steel, cobalt- and titanium-base alloys [3]. Stainless steels are now primarily reserved for trauma therapy devices, such as intramedullary nails, plates and screws, etc., with partial and total joint replacement applications dominated by the latter two alloy systems.

Even retrieved contemporary devices show evidence of metal loss and metallosis still occasionally occurs in implant sites. This has led to a renewed study of *in vivo* corrosion and wear processes. All of the alloys in general use today are highly corrosion and resistant in engineering terms and most are also highly wear resistant. However, their use in total joint replacements devices, such as metal/polymer articulating THRs, produces chronic elevations of serum, and in some cases urine, content of various metals by two- to five-fold over normal levels [8]. Thus, there is a continuing need for a general inquiry into the biological effects of implanted metallic devices.

Beginning in the 1960's, this inquiry has focused on answering four questions. These questions, with brief summaries of their answers to date, are:
1. *What and how much is released from an implant?* All metal implants release metal. Release rates by corrosion and wear processes are fairly modest, except in the presence of device loosening. Fracture of devices, deliberate modularity and metal/metal articulations all increase release rates significantly.
2. *What are the chemical and physical forms?* Metal is released as ions bound to organic molecules, as solid and colloidal particles and as precipitates. There are essentially no free metallic ions. However, there remains uncertainty about the chemical valence of metallic moieties in some complexed forms.
3. *How are they distributed, stored, and excreted?* Each soluble metallic species has a different characteristic distribution, storage and excretion pattern. Some metals, such as cobalt, are excreted rapidly and do not accumulate; others, such as chromium, collect in local tissues and remote sites, such as the liver and the kidney.
4. *What are the biological consequences?* With the exception of iron and chromium, little is still known about the metabolic fate of metals released at low, chronic rates from implants. We must continue to rely on fundamental studies of biological effects of pure metals and free ions.

It can be fairly said, in summary, that we now have a great deal of knowledge concerning the first question, some information concerning the second and third and are just beginning to appreciate the magnitude of the issues raised by the fourth question.

Metallic Biomaterials

When we examine the roster of alloys in general use today (Table **1**), we can summarize the composition of these materials as follows:
   Three elements constitute the basis of these alloy systems: Fe (Iron) in the stainless steels, Ti

Table 1 ASTM standards for metallic biomaterials [1]

Stainless Steels (Iron-Base):	
F 138	Specification for Stainless Steel Bar and Wire for Surgical Implants (Special Quality)
F 745	Specification for 18 Chromium-12.5 Nickel-2.5 Molybdenum Stainless Steel for Cast and Solution-Annealed Surgical Implant Applications
F 1314	Specification for Wrought Nitrogen Strengthened, High Manganese, High Chromium Stainless Steel Bar and Wire for Surgical Implants
F 1586	Specification for Wrought Nitrogen Strengthened-21 Chromium-10 Nickel-3 Manganese-2.5 Molybdenum Stainless Steel Bar for Surgical Implants
Titanium/Titanium-Base Alloys:	
F 67	Specification for Unalloyed Titanium for Surgical Implant Applications
F 136	Specification for Wrought Titanium 6Al-4 V ELI Alloy for Surgical Implant Applications
F 1295	Specification for Wrought Titanium-6 Aluminum-7 Niobium Alloy for Surgical Implant Applications
F 1713	Specification for Wrought Titanium-13 Niobium-13 Zirconium Alloy for Surgical Implant Applications
Cobalt-Base Alloys:	
F 75	Specification for Cast Cobalt-Chromium-Molybdenum Alloy for Surgical Implant Applications
F 90	Specification for Wrought Cobalt-Chromium-Tungsten- Nickel Alloy for Surgical Implant Applications
F 562	Specification for Wrought Cobalt-35 Nickel-20 Chromium-10 Molybdenum Alloy for Surgical Implant Applications
F 563	Specification for Wrought Cobalt-Nickel-Chromium-Molybdenum Tungsten-Iron Alloy for Surgical Implant Applications
F 961	Specification for Cobalt-Nickel-Chromium-Molybdenum Alloy Forgings for Surgical Implant Applications
F 1058	Specification for Wrought Cobalt-Chromium-Nickel-Molybdenum-Iron Alloy for Surgical Implant Applications
F 1537	Specification for Wrought Cobalt-28 Chromium-6 Molybdenum Alloy for Surgical Implants
Other metals and alloys:	
F 560	Specification for Unalloyed Tantalum for Surgical Implant Applications

(Titanium) in the titanium base alloys and Co (Cobalt) in the cobalt base so-called "super alloys."

Nine additional metallic elements are present as deliberately added alloying elements: Al (Aluminum), Cr (Chromium), Mn (Manganese), Mo (Molybdenum), Nb (Niobium), Ni (Nickel), Ta (Tantalum), V (Vanadium) and W (Tungsten). These elements are used, in various proportions, to provide the desired chemical resistance and mechanical properties for each application.

Typical examples of each alloy system, with compositions in weight percent, are [1]:

- Stainless steel:
  F-1314: 22 Cr, 12.5 Ni, 5 Mn,
  2.5 Mo (balance) Fe
- Titanium base:
  F-136: 6 Al 4 V (balance) Ti
- Cobalt base:
  F-1537: 28 Cr, 6 Mo,
  (< 1) Ni, (balance) Co

Biological Response

Considerations of the biological implications of the elemental composition of implants can be grouped under four general headings:

- *Metabolic:* Does the element have a normal concentration dependent biological role?
- *Bacteriologic:* Does the element play a role in initiation, promotion or defense against infection?
- *Immunologic:* Does the element play a role in enabling or mounting specific immune system responses?
- *Carcinogenic:* Does the element play a role in initiation or promotion of neoplastic transformation?

Table 2 summarizes what is known about metallic alloy elemental components in regard to these four considerations.
Note carefully two points:
- The information in this table is drawn from a variety of sources and is dervied primarily from human workplace exposure and animal toxicology. Biological effects depend upon chemical form and valence, as well as dose and dose rate. Unfortunately, as previously suggested, little is still known about the biological effects of the exact forms and doses of metal bearing species encountered in association with chronic human implants.
- Toxicological research is usually performed in animals with soluble forms and compounds.

The role that metallic particles play in biological response to chronic implants has been discussed elsewhere [4,12]. Apart from recognizing that the production of small metallic debris, such as the submicron wear debris shed by metal/metal articulations, has an indirect effect of radically increasing the availability of soluble forms [8], we shall not further discuss response to such solid forms.

Examination of Table 1, in which the three alloy bases are highlighted for emphasis, reveals that our concerns lie primarily with immunologic and carcinogenic effects.

With regard to immunologic responses, it is now well recognized that certain metallic elements, in our case, Co, Cr, Ni and possibly V, may combine with native proteins to form haptenic complexes capable, in animal models, of enabling or mounting type IV delayed hypersensitivity reactions. Careful evaluation of patients, with and without chronic metallic implants reveals, in any study group, some proportion of sensitive individuals, and within that subgroup, a smaller proportion who show signs of immune response, as indicated by reduced leukocyte chemotactic ability, in the presence of the appropriate haptenic complex.

With a colleague, we have recently made an analysis of published reports of sensitivity associated with THR arthroplasty [6]. When studies are performed using *in vitro* leukocyte tests, such as the leukocyte inhibitory factor (LIF) test [7], one can draw the following conclusions:

In the general (non-symptomatic) population (N = 500), individuals have a 10% mean risk of being sensitive to one or more of Co, Cr or Ni (range: 8 – 14%).

Among patients with well-functioning implants, of various alloy compositions (8 studies, N = 888), individuals have a 25% mean risk of being sensitive to one or more of Co, Cr or Ni (study range: 3 – 43%).

Among patients with implants, of various alloy compositions, that have failed for various reasons (5 studies, N = 251), individuals have a 50% mean risk of being sensitive to one or more of Co, Cr or Ni (study range: 13 – 69%).

From this analysis, we draw the following tentative conclusions:
- Metallic alloys used in prostheses contain and release known human immunogens.
- Risk is related to exposure and exposure duration.
- Sensitivity is not generally related to clinical symptoms.

Table 2 Biological response to elemental components of metallic biomaterials

	Al	Co	Cr	Fe	Mn	Mo	Nb	Ni	Ta	Ti	V	W
Metabolic	Y	Y	Y	Y	?	?	N	Y	N	?	N	?
Bacteriologic	N	N	N	Y	N	N	N	N	N	N	N	N
Immunologic	N	Y	Y	N	N	N	N	Y	N	N	?	N
Carcinogenic	N	Y	Y	N	?	N	N	Y	N	?	?	N

Key: Y = Yes, N = No, ? = Unknown/uncertain

With regard to the last point, it must be emphasized that only in rare individual cases is it possible to make a link between sensitivity and symptoms or clinical outcome of an arthroplasty procedure. We do not suggest that prospective testing for THR and TKR candidates is indicated at this time, except in the presence of a history of metal "allergy." Even if such testing indicates Ni sensitivity, there is still a choice possible between titanium- and cobalt-base alloys, as F-1537, the most commonly used super alloy, is essentially nickel free.

With regard to carcinogenic responses, it is now accepted that certain metallic elements, in our case, Co, Cr, Ni and possibly Mn, Ti and V, are carcinogenic or are capable of forming at least one carcinogenic compound. Of these, only Co, Cr and Ni are classified as presumptive human carcinogens [2].

Although there are now more than 25 case reports of primary implant site tumors associated with total joint replacement arthroplasty [11], our concern has always been focused more on the possibility of increased risk of systemic (e.g. circulatory system) or remote site neoplastic transformation.

There have now been three epidemiological studies of cancer incidence after THR [5,9,13] and one after TKR arthroplasty [10], covering in all over 50,000 patients and 400,000 patient years. Overall risk of neoplasia is not significantly elevated; however, there appears to be an association of elevated risk of leukemia/lymphoma with the use the McKee-Farrar THR, an early design with a metal/metal articulation,

From these reports, we draw the following tentative conclusions:
- Metallic alloys used in chronic implants contain and release presumptive human carcinogens.
- Risk is related to exposure and exposure duration. (Human latency for chemical carcinogenesis increases with decreasing dose rate and is generally about 20 years in duration.)
- Clinical evidence suggests that, while risk may be real, it is probably small for patients with less than 20 years life expectancy.
- Care should still be exercised in the use of stainless steels and cobalt-base super alloys in high surface area and/or high wear rate designs in younger patients.

Conclusions

In conclusion, it is fair to state that metallic alloys in use today in chronic implants are generally safe and effective, and evoke minimal unintended biological responses. However, our knowledge base of actual, statistically valid data about clinical incidence and prevalence of adverse biomaterials-related outcomes remains woefully inadequate. Therefore, it is advisable to exercise care in the use of high metal release rate designs, such as ones with excessive modularity or metal/metal articulations, especially in younger, more active patients.

Acknowledgment

Preparation of this article was supported by NIH grant AR 39310. General support from Zimmer, Inc and The Rush Arthritis and Orthopaedics Institute is also gratefully recognized.

References

1. Annual Standards Book of ASTM Standards, Vol. 13.01: Medical Devices; Emergency Medical Services. West Conshocken: Amer. Soc. Testing Materials, 1999
2. Black J: Biological Performance of Materials: Fundamentals of Biocompatibility, 3rd. ed. New York: Marcel Dekker, p. 241, 1999
3. Black J: Biomaterials in total hip arthroplasty – Overview. In: The Adult Hip, Rubash H, Callaghan J, Rosenberg A (eds), Philadelphia: Lippincott-Raven, p. 87, 1997
4. Black J, Jacobs JJ: Effect of Material on Long-term Survivorship. in: Revision Total Hip Arthroplasty, Steinberg ME, Garino JP (eds), Philadelphia: Lippincott-Raven, p. 73, 1998
5. Gillespie, WJ, Frampton, CMA, Henderson, RJ et al.: The incidence of cancer following total hip replacement. J. Bone Joint Surg. 70 B: 539–42, 1988
6. Hallab N, Jacobs JJ, Black J: Hypersensitivity Associated with Metallic Biomaterials. In: Biomaterials Engineering and Devices: Human Applications, Wise DL (ed), New York: Humana Press (in press, 2000)
7. Hallab NJ, Jacobs JJ, Black J: Hypersensitivity to metallic biomaterials: A review of leukocyte migration inhibition assays. Biomaterials (in press, 2000)

8 Jacobs JJ, Skipor AK, Doorn PF, et al.: Cobalt and chromium concentrations in patients with metal-on-metal total hip replacements. Clin. Orthop. Rel. Res. 329 S: S256–S263, 1996
9 Nyrén O, McLaughlin JK, Gridley G et al.: Cancer risk after total hip replacement with metal implants. J. Natl. Cancer Inst. 87: 28–33, 1995
10 Paavolainen P, Pukkala E, Pulkkinen P et al.: Cancer incidence after total knee arthroplasty. Acta Ortop. Scand. 70: 609–17, 1999
11 Rock, MG: Cancer. in Handbook of Biomaterial Properties, J Black, GW Hastings (eds), London: Chapman and Hall, p. 529, 1998
11 Shanbhag AS, Jacobs JJ, Black J et al: Effects of particles on fibroblast proliferation and bone resorption *in vitro*. Clin. Orthop. Rel. Res. 342: 205–217, 1997
13 Visuri Y, Koskenvuo M: Cancer risk after McKee-Farrar total hip replacement. Orthop. 14: 137–142, 1991

3.5 Allergological Aspects of Implant Biocompatibility

P. Thomas, Munich, Germany

Introduction

After implantation the immunological biocompatibility of a given material is described in terms of acute and chronic inflammatory responses of the host. The initial surgical procedure to implant the foreign material by itself will generate an acute inflammation. The intensity and duration of this response are related to factors like the immunogenicity of components of the devices, the different anatomical sites of implantation and the reactive capacity of the organism. Besides the vast majority of patients with normal wound healing, osseointegration or fibrous capsule formation, some individuals with hypersensitivity reactions have been reported. In association with metallic implants localized or hematogenous, generalized eczema, local swelling or recurrent urticaria have been described (2,3,17). Aseptic loosening is discussed to be partly due to immunological/allergic mechanisms (2,11). However, it is even an open question, to which degree in already sensitised patients the implantation of the relevant metals may provoke complications. This is reflected by only few patients showing complications in contrast to the nickel, cobalt or chromium sensitisation rates in the general population. With the restriction of different study populations (age, sex, lifestyle) cutaneous sensitisation rates to one or more of those metals are estimated to range between 2–10% (10,24,33). In addition, it is under discussion, how to prove the link between intolerance of implanted devices and contact allergy to one of their components proven by patch test.

Mechanisms

According to Coombs and Gell hypersensitivity reactions are classified into four types (14): Type I to III reactions are antibody mediated; examples are immediate reactions like urticaria or rhinoconjunctivitis, furthermore cytotoxic antibody reactions and immune complex formation with complement induced inflammation. Type IV reactions (delayed type) to low molecular weight substances are T-cell mediated coinvolving macrophages or eosinophils in the inflammatory response. They include contact dermatitis or pseudolymphoma formation due to Nickel or chromium/cobalt.

Several conditions may favor the induction of hypersensitivity reactions:

The immunogenic/allergenic potency of a given substance. This is often linked with its capacity to provoke irritation or to penetrate the (muco)cutaneous barrier. Examples of contact allergens with such properties are not polymerized acrylates or preservatives like isothiazolones (15). Direct effects of high nickel or cobalt load are rather immunosuppressive or toxic. However, low exposure may directly induce expression of adhesion molecules on vascular endothelium thus favoring recruitment of proinflammatory cells into the tisssue (8). With regard to metal recognition by T-cells it has been speculated that nickel (hapten) modified proteins are "seen" by the T-cell receptor (TCR) in the context of MHC class II molecules (31). A high density of TCR-ligands, as generated on the surface of antigen presenting cells by haptens like nickel, would preferentially induce a TH1-response. This leads to production of IFN-γ and TNF-α, typical mediators of delayed type hypersensitivity.

Properties of implant materials. The release of potential allergens like nickel, chromium or cobalt depends on composition, surface modification, chemical and physical corrosion factors. Low pH and low oxygenation of adjacent tissue may influence metallic surface – even leading to titanium release in surrounding tissue (40). Nickel and cobalt ions are thought to be rapidly transported from the implant site and eliminated in the urine. When contained in particulate debris or in the case of chromium-cobalt wear, persistance in the tissue is often observed (20). Whereas the tribological behaviour of bioceramics is reported to minimize the wear rate (41), articulating surfaces depending on different other material combinations are linked with more or less wear formation. Amount, composition and size of different particulate species will lead to a varying degree of macrophage, fibroblast and osteoblast response (1,9,27,29,30,39,42). The macrophage reaction to the particle load, beeing phagocytosable or not, includes production of IL-6, TNF-α and PGE$_2$, creating an inflammatory bone-resorbing environment. It is still unclear, to which extent specific T-cellular sensitisation is favored in this environment.

The tissue environment. In the mucocutaneous range impaired barrier function (prexisting eczema, area of leg ulcer, semicovered dental implants) or occlusion (wearing gloves, intertriginous areas) facilitate antigen penetration and sensitisation. The ease of sensitisation seems to differ between various organs, the skin and subcutaneous range beeing most susceptible. This is partly due to the influence of organ specific immune control like SALT (skin associated lymphoid tissue) or MALT (mucosa associated lymphoid tissue). In addition, the differential expression of homing receptors may – in the case of systemic responses – induce preferential accumulation of circulating specific T-cells.

Adjuvans factors. Proinflammatory effects are mediated by particles or microbial constituents like liposaccharide or DNA fragments, macrophages beeing one of the target cells (28). Due to other preexisting allergic sensitisations peri-/postoperative inflammation may develop and facilitate sensitisation to implant constituents. Examples are allergic reactions to disinfectants, to antibiotics or natural rubber latex.

Patient derived factors. Atopic individuals are characterized by a genetically determined tendency to develop diseases like allergic rhinoconjunctivitis, asthma or atopic eczema. The irritable skin is often a typical feature. A genetical susceptibility for metal allergy or for development of delayed type or granulomatous foreign body reactions is discussed by some authors (22,23). The influence of preexisting metal allergy will be discussed below.

Clinical Manifestation

Among the individuals with dermatitis due to proven metal contact allergy, about 10% experience recurrence or aggravation of skin disease by "internal allergen exposure". The existance of this so called systemically induced contact dermatitis has been reproducibly proven by oral challenge studies (16,37). Underlying characteristics of these patients are identified only in part (34). A source of exposure may not only be alimentary uptake but also metal release from implanted devices. There are several clinical reports of eczema reactions, both local and remote, to metallic implants (5,13,17,19,38). Figure 1 shows a patient with a well tolerated titanium-based hip endoprothesis, but local eczema and loosening of a cobalt-chromium based knee endoprosthesis. Allergological diagnostics revealed a chromate contact allergy and a type I sensitisation to natural rubber latex.

It is difficult to estimate the actual incidence of allergic responses to implanted metallic devices that contribute to patient morbidity and to impairment of the implant function. Whereas case reports show patients with local or systemic intolerance reactions (21), in larger study populations low incidence of allergy-mediated cutaneous or orthopedic complications are reported (6,17,26). Carlsson and Möller for example retrospectively examined patients with contact allergy to metals proven before implantation of metallic devices (4) Out of the 39 patients one had developed exzema of the feet and papular itching eruption of the trunk, both subsiding only after removal of the osteosynthesis material used to treat an ankle fracture. Beeing deceased at the time of retrospective analysis, this patient like others could not be included. Out of the 18 remaining patients three had developed eczema reactions, but also had preexisting eczema. In two patients mechanical loosening of the implanted devices was seen. Some patients even showed no more cutaneous reactivity upon renewed skin testing at the time of follow-up. Thus, as conclusion an overall good implant tolerance was reported.

This study is reflecting some of the problems during analysis of suspected immunological intolerance of implants:
- Skin testing is a standard procedure, but may not necessarily reflect reactivity of other or-

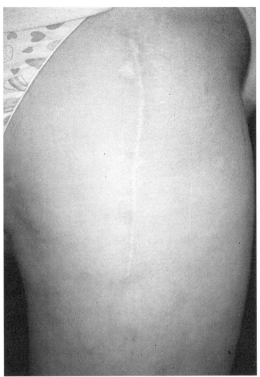 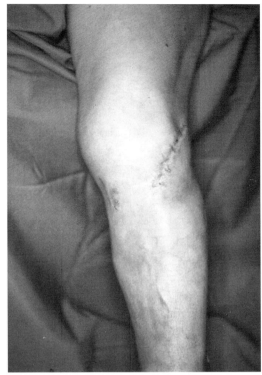

Fig. 1 **a** Well tolerated titanium-based hip endoprothesis and **b** eczematous reaction with loosening at the site of a cobalt-chromium based knee-endoprothesis in the same patient (with chromate allergy).

gans and may vary with the patients overall reactivity.
- Unusual manifestations of allergic reactions may not always be recognized as such (12, 43).
- Additional analysis of the periimplantar tissue or peripheral blood cell reactivity can not always be performed.
- It is not completely clear, under which conditions tolerance to local or systemic metal exposure can be favored (36).

Immune responses that compromise the acceptability of an implanted device, are often seen under the picture of periimplantar macrophage activation (especially wear-associated) or as lympho-histiocytic infiltrates (Fig. 2). In order to further evaluate their functional characteristics, molecular biology techniques can be applied. In the case of a patient with implant loosening and local discomfort, the demonstration of periimplantar oligoclonal (antigen-driven) T-cell infiltrate together with Th1-type mediator production helped to link the intolerance to a proven dichromate allergy (35). With regard to clinical allergological diagnostics, history and clinical picture are supplemented by epicutaneous testing. The testwise subcutaneous implantation of aliquots of the material in question is still under discussion. Since standards are missing, it is not clear, wether this procedure may enhance sensitisation or if it allows conclusions with regard to the future implantation site. In vitro methods like lymphocyte activation assays are so far restricted to academic approach (32).

Outlook

Implant materials will be used increasingly and for a growing number of applications. Sometimes immunological interactions with the host are only seen after long term persistence in the organism, as reflected by the ongoing discussion regarding silicone-based breast implants. It is evi-

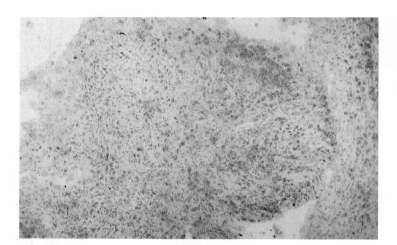

Fig. 2 Periimplantar T-cellular infiltrate (immunohistology with anti-CD3-antibody). Cobalt-chromium osteosynthesis material; patient with chromate allergy [from (35)].

dent, that components of most implants can be released into the tissue (7,18,20,25). However, the different interactions with the biological system are not always completely understood.

With regard to immunological-allergological biocompatibility, an interdisciplinary approach including cellular and molecular biology in vitro and clinical follow up will help to optimize implant materials and to identify patient derived predisposing conditions.

Literature

1. Akatsu T, Takahashi N, Udagawa N, Imamura K, Yamaguchi A, Sato K, Nagata N, Suda T (1991) Role of prostaglandins in interleukin-1-induced bone resorption in mice in vitro. J Bone Miner Res 6: 183–190
2. Black J (1999) Allergic foreign body response In: Biological performance of materials – fundamentals of biocompatibility, 3 d ed., Marcel Dekker New York, Basel: 215–232
3. Carlsson A, Magnussen B, Möller H (1980) Metal sensitivity in patients with metal to plastic total hip arthroplasties. Acta Orthop Scand 51: 57–62
4. Carlsson A, Möller H (1989) Implantation of orthopaedic devices in patients with metal allergy. Acta Derm Venereol 69: 62–66
5. Cramers M, Lucht L (1977) Metal sensitivity in patients treated for tibial fractures with plates of stainless steel. Acta Orthop Scand 48: 245–249
6. Duchna HW, Nowack U, Merget R, Muhr G, Schultze-Werninghaus G (1998) Prospektive Untersuchung zur Bedeutung der Kontaktsensibilisierung durch Metallimplantate. Zentralbl Chir 123: 1271–1276
7. Fischer-Brandies E, Zeintl W, Schramel P, Benner KU (1992) Zum Nachweis von Titan im Organismus bei temporärer Alloplastik. Dtsch Zahnärztl Z 47: 526–528
8. Goebeler M, Meinarddus-Hager G, Roth J, Goerdt S, Sorg C (1993) Nickel Chloride and Cobalt Chloride, two common contact sensitizers, directly induce expression of intercellular adhesion molecule-1 (ICAM-1), vascular cell adhesion molecule-1 (VCAM-1), and endothelial leukocyte adhesion molecule (ELAM-1) by endothelial cells. J Invest Dermatol 100(6): 759–765
9. Glant TT, Jacobs JJ, Molnar G, Shanbhag AS, Valyon M, Galante JO (1993) Bone resorption activity of particulate-stimulated macrophages. J Bone Miner Res 8: 1071–1079
10. Goh CL (1985) Prevalence of contact allergy by sex, race and age. Contact Dermatitis 14: 237–240
11. Goodman SB (1996) Does the immune system play a role in loosening and osteolysis of total joint replacements? J Long Term Eff Med Implants 6(2): 91–101
12. Hayashi K, Kaneko H, Kawachi S, Saida T (1999) Allergic contact dermatitis and osteomyelitis due to sternal stainless steel wire. Contact Dermatitis 41: 115–116
13. Hildebrand HF, Veron C, Martin P (1988) In: Hildebrandt HF, Champy M (eds.) Biocompatibility of Co-Cr-Ni-alloys. Plenum press, New York: 201–211
14. Janeway CA, Travers P, Walport M, Capra JD (eds.) (1999) Immunobiology: the immune system in health and disease, 4th ed., Elsevier Science Ltd., London: 461–488

15 Kanerva L, Tarvainen K, Pinola A, Leino T, Granlund H, Estlander T, Jolanki R, Förström L 1994) A single accidental exposure may result in a chemical burn, primary sensitization and allergic contact dermatitis. Contact Dermatitis 31: 229–235
16 Klaschka F, Ring J (1990) Systemically induced (hematogenous) contact eczema. Seminars in Dermatology 9: 210–215
17 Kubba R, Taylor JS, Marks KE (1981) Cutaneous complications of orthopedic implants. Arch Dermatol 117: 554–560
18 Levenson T, Greenberger PA, Murphy R (1996) Peripheral blood eosinophilia, hyper-immunoglobulinemia A and fatigue: possible complications following rupture of silicone breast implants. Ann Allergy Asthma Immunol 77(2): 119–122
19 Mayor MB, Merritt K, Brown SA (1980) Metal allergy and the surgical patient. Am J Surg 139: 477–479
20 Merritt K, Brown S (1996) Distribution of cobalt chromium wear and corrosion products and biologic reactions. Clin Orthop Rel Res 329: S233–S243
21 Meyrick TRH, Rademaker M, Goddard NJ, Munro DD (1987) Severe eczema of the hands due to an orthopaedic plate made of Vitallium. Br Med J 294: 106–107
22 Mitchison NA (1992) Specialisation, tolerance, memory, competition, latency, and strife among T-cells. Ann Rev Immunol 10: 1–12
23 Mozzanica N, Rizzolo L, Veneroni G, Diotti R, Hepeisen S, Finzi AF (1990) HLA-A, B, C and DR antigens in nickel contact sensitivity. Brit J Dermatol 122: 309–313
24 Möller H (1990) Nickel dermatitis: problems solved and unsolved. Contact Dermatitis 23: 217–220
25 Pathak YV, Vanmeeteren R, Dwivedi C (1996) Aluminum polymeric implants: in vitro – in vivo evaluations. J Biomater Appl 11: 62–75
26 Rakoski J, von Mayenburg J, Düngemann H, Borelli S (1986) Metallallergien bei Patienten mit Metallimplantaten im Knochen. Allergologie 9: 160–163
27 Rodgers K, Klykken P, Jacobs J, Frondoza C, Tomazic V, Zelikoff J (1997) Immunotoxicity of medical devices. Fundam Appl Toxicol 36: 1–14
28 Scott P, Trinchieri G (1997) IL-12 as an adjuvant for cell mediated immunity. Semin Immunol 9: 285–291
29 Shanbhag AS, Jacobs JJ, Glant TT, Gilbert JL, Black J, Galante JO (1994) Composition and morphology of wear debris in failed uncemented total hip replacement arthroplasty. J Bone Joint Surg B 76: 60–67
30 Shanbhag AS, Jacobs JJ, Black J, Galante JO, Glant TT (1995) Cellular mediators secreted by interfacial membranes obtained at revision total hip arthroplasty. J Arthroplasty 10: 498–506
31 Sinigaglia F (1994) The molecular basis of metal recognition by T cells. J Invest Dermatol 102: 398–401
32 Summer B, Thomas P, Przybilla B, Sander CA (1999) Molecular analysis of T-cell clonality and with concomitant specific T-cell proliferation in vitro in nickel-allergic individuals. Allergy 54, Suppl 52: 8 (A)
33 Thomas P, Meurer M (1996) Immunopathien der Haut. In: Medizinische Immunologie (Hrsg Baenkler HW), Ecomed Verlag Landsberg, Kapitel III: 1–96
34 Thomas P, Holz T, Messer G, Przybilla B (1999) Nickel allergic patients with or without reactions upon oral nickel challenge: lymphocyte reactivity and cytokine pattern. J Allergy Clin Immunol 103: 85 (A)
35 Thomas P, Thomas M, Summer B, Naumann T, Sander CA, Przybilla B (2000) Intolerance of osteosynthesis material: evidence of dichromate contact allergy with concomitant oligoclonal T-cell infiltrate and Th1-type cytokine expression in the periimplantar tissue. Allergy, in press
36 Van Hoogstraten I, Boos C, Boden D, von Blomberg ME, Scheper RJ, Kraal G (1993) Oral induction of tolerance to nickel sensitization in mice. J Invest Dermatol 101: 26–31
37 Veien NK, Hattel T, Laurberg G (1994) Chromate allergic patients challenged orally with potassium dichromate. Contact Dermatitis 31: 137–139
38 Waterman AH, Schrik JJ (1985) Allergy in hip arthroplasty. Contact Dermatitis 13: 294–301
39 Willert HG, Semlitsch M (1996) Tissue reactions to plastic and metallic wear products. Clin Orthop Rel Res 333: 4–14
40 Willert HG, Broback LG, Buchhorn GH, Köster G, Lang I, Ochsner P, Schenk R (1996) Crevice corrosion of cemented titanium alloy stems in total hip replacements. Clin Orthop Rel Res 333: 51–75
41 Willmann G (2000) Bioceramics in orthopaedics: what did we learn in 25 years? Med Orth Tech 120: 10–16
42 Yao J, Glant TT, Lark MW, Mikecz K, Jacobs JJ, Hutchinson NI, Hoerrner LA, Kuettner KE, Galante JO (1995) The potential role of fibroblasts in periprosthetic osteolysis. Fibroblast response to titanium particulates. J Bone Miner Res 10: 1417–1427
43 Zemtsov A, Cameron GS, Montalvo-Lugo V (1997) Nickel-induced lymphocytoma cutis of the earlobe. Contact Dermatitis 36: 266

4 Advanced Materials for Bearing Surfaces in Joint Replacement

4.1 Simulator Testing of the Wear Couple ZTA-on-Polyethylene

A. Toni, S. Affatato, B. Bordini

Introduction

Ceramic materials, alumina and zirconia, has been widely used as bearing material of hip prosthetic devices since their introduction more than 20 years ago [1,2]. Among the ceramics, alumina is probably the most commonly used material. Some authors suggest that the use of zirconia may improve the mechanical strength of the prosthetic head over alumina [3], while others state that zirconia may also reduce polyethylene wear with respect to alumina [4,6].

Pure zirconia heads were compared to pure alumina ones and two types of mixed oxides ceramic heads (alumina and respectively 60% and 80% of zirconia) in terms of wear behaviour against UHMW-Polyethylene in a hip joint simulator with bovine calf serum.

Materials and Methods

Ultra-high-molecular-weight polyethylene acetabular cups (ETO gas irradiated), including four soaked control cups in order to evaluate the effect of fluid sorption, were tested against pure zirconia (Zr, AmZirOx [Astro Met Inc., OHIO, USA]), 32 mm balls, pure alumina (Al, Biolox [CeramTec, Germany]), 32 mm balls, and two type of experimental mixed-oxide ceramics with different percentage of alumina and zirconia, 32 mm balls (60% Zr + 40% Al = mixed#1; 80% Zr + 20% Al = mixed#2).

The eight mixed-oxides heads were manufactured in-house. The manufacturing process was developed by Centro Ceramico (Bologna – Italy) and by FN S.p.A. (Bosco Marengo – Italy).

The study was carried out using a twelve stations hip joint wear simulator (Shore Western, U.S.A.). In each station the implants were mounted in non anatomical position (upside down): the disadvantage of the non anatomical position, as accumulation of the third body particles on the sliding distance, has been solved applied a test procedure that included periodic washing and cleaning of the specimens every 500,000 cycles. The whole test lasted 5,000,000 cycles, which represent a clinical follow-up of approximately five years [7].

The heads were mounted using self-aligning connection components while the cups were fixed to a polyurethane holder and mounted on a bearing block to represent the natural flexion angle between cup and hip joint load axis. The stations were filled with lubricant in order to wet completely the specimen's contact surfaces. The lubricant used was 30% sterile bovine calf serum (SIGMA, St. Louis, USA) and 70% deionised water plus 0.2% sodium azide (E. Merck, Darmstadt, Germany) to retard bacterial degradation during the wear test.

The load profile was sinusoidal with a max force of about 2 KN and a frequency of 1 Hz. The acetabular cups were removed from the simulator every 500,000 cycles, and cleaned at each stop-weight measurement. The test was restarted with fresh serum solution. The cups were cleaned using a special detergent called Clean 70 (Elma GmbH, Germany) to remove dust and possible particles debris in an ultrasonic bath maintained at 20 °C for 10 minutes. After rinsing the cups were put back in the ultrasonic bath with deionised water for an additional 15 minutes. The cups were then dried with nitrogen gas. During any interruption of the test, the cups were stored in a closed, dust-free container at 70% of relative humidity.

In the present work polyethylene wear was calculated by the weight loss method using a microbalance (SARTORIUS AG, Germany) with a sensitivity of 0.01 mg and an uncertainty of ± 0.10 mg.

Each weight measurement was repeated for three times and the average weight was used for

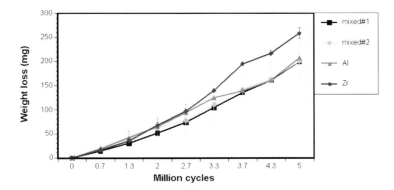

Fig. 1 Cumulative weight loss up to 5 million cycles.

calculations. The test and soak-cup controls were treated identically in order to obtain the same exposure to the wash, rinse and drying fluids.

Results

Due to a mechanical problem (head failure), one of the pure alumina specimens had to be stopped after 2.7 million cycles; the other specimens completed the planned five million cycles.

After five million cycles the total measured wear of the polyethylene cups for the four types of ceramic heads was 200 ± 45 mg (mixed#2), 201 ± 36 mg (mixed#1) and 260 ± 11 mg (Zr); the remaining pure alumina specimen wore 210 mg of polyethylene. The evolution of cumulative weight loss of all polyethylene acetabular cups is plotted in Fig. 1.

None of these differences were statistically significant (Kruskall-Wallis nonparametric test) but, owing to the samples small dimension, the obtained results could be unreliable.

The wear rate was calculated with two separate regressions over the 0.0 – 2.7 million cycles and the 3.3 – 5.0 million cycles spans when the specimens tend to wear in, Fig. 2. Polyethylene specimens coupled with pure alumina, showed in the first 2.7 million cycles an average wear rate of 37 ± 6 mg/cycles × 10^6 (average ± standard error of the mean) and polyethylene specimens coupled with pure zirconia specimens 41 ± 2 mg/cycles × 10^6. Polyethylene specimens coupled with the mixed-oxides specimens showed a lower wear rate: 30 ± 5 mg/cycles × 10^6 and 30 ± 3 mg/cycles × 10^6 for the mixed#1 and mixed#2, respectively.

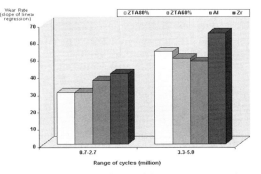

Fig. 2 Wear Rate as slope of linear regression (0 – 2.7 vs. 3.3 – 5 million cycles).

Between 3.3 and 5.0 million cycles the polyethylene acetabular cup coupled with the remaining pure alumina specimen had an average wear rate of 48 mg/cycles × 10^6. The other specimens showed an average wear rate of 50 ± 12 mg/cycles × 10^6 (mixed#1), 54 ± 13 mg/cycles × 10^6 (mixed#2) and 65 ± 7 mg/cycles × 10^6 (Zr).

Discussion

It is still controversial as to whether alumina femoral heads or zirconia femoral heads are more advantageous when articulating against UHMW-Polyethylene acetabular cups.

It is a fact that the wear rate of ceramics (alumina or zirconia) articulating against UHMW-Polyethylene is lower than the wear rate of metal ball heads [2,8,9].

The results presented here clearly demonstrate the influence of the zirconia content on the tribologic behaviour using a hip joint wear simulator. Our results, obtained in a hip joint simulator, emphasised that the experimental ceramic heads with less percentage of zirconia (mixed#1) demonstrated a better wear behaviour than the experimental ceramic heads with more percentage of zirconia (mixed#2). Wear couples generating high wear rate consist of pure zirconia specimens. However, the experimental results did not show significant difference between the two experimental ceramic materials or in comparison with pure materials. All specimens, regardless of the material, had the same level of surface roughness.

This was the first study to validate the influence of zirconia percentage in ceramic femoral heads. Zirconia ceramics needs additives such as calcia (CaO), magnesia (MgO) and/or yttria in order to stabilise the material in either the tetragonal or the cubic phase [10]. However, composite of alumina-zirconia system can be prepared without any additives to stabilise the zirconia and in order to obtain a material that present higher toughness values inducing higher wear resistance. Such material could be zirconia toughened alumina (ZTA). Liang (1990) [11] has shown that an addition of 5% of zirconia was very efficient in increasing crack resistance of alumina and decrease of crack velocities of several order of magnitude. Chevalier et al. (1999) [12] in their study demonstrated that the addition of zirconia particles increases crack resistance. Further studies are needed to address this issue.

References

1 Kaddicck C, Pfaff HG (1999) Wear study in the Alumina-zirconia system. In: Sedel L, Willmann G (eds.) Reliability and Long-Term Results of Ceramics in Orthopaedics. 4th International CeramTec Symposium, Germany, pp 96–101
2 Willmann G, Fruh HJ, Pfaff HG. Wear characteristics of sliding pairs of zirconia (Y-TZP) for hip endoprostheses. Biomaterials 1996; 17(22): 2157–2162
3 Cuckler JM, Bearcroft J, Asgian CM. Femoral head technologies to reduce polyethylene wear in total hip arthroplasty. Clinical Orthopaedics and Related Research 1995; 317: 57–63
4 Kumar P, Oka M, Ukeuchi K, Shimizu K. Low Wear Rate Of Uhmwpe Aginst Zirconia Ceramic (Y-Psz) In Comparison To Alumina Ceramic And Sus 316 Alloy. Journal of Biomedical Materials Research 1991; 25: 813–828
5 Toni A, Terzi S, Sudanese A, Tabarroni M, Zappoli FA, Stea S, Giunti A. The use of ceramic in prosthetic hip surgery. The state of the art. Chir. Organi Mov. 1995; 80: 13–25
6 MCKellop H, Lu B, Benya P (1992). Friction, lubrication and wear of cobalt-chromium, alumina and zirconia hip prostheses compared on a joint simulator. 38th Annual Meeting, Orthopaedic Research Society, Washington D. C., 402
7 Saikko VO. Wear of the polyethylene acetabular cups against alumina femoral heads. Acta Orthop Scand 1993; 64 (5): 507–512
8 Oonishi H, Amino H, Ueno M, Yunoki H 1999 Concepts and designs with Ceramics for Total Hip and Knee Replacement. In: Sedel L, Willmann G (eds.) Reliability and Long-Term Results of Ceramics in Orthopaedics. 4th International CeramTec Symposium, Germany, 7–28
9 Goossens M (1999) The Transcend Alumina Ceramic Hip Articulation System. In: Sedel L, Willmann G (eds.) Reliability and Long-Term Results of Ceramics in Orthopaedics. 4th International CeramTec Symposium, Germany, 29–32
10 Li J, Hastings GW (1999) Oxide bioceramics: inert ceramic materials in medicine and dentistry. In: Black J, Hastings G (eds.) Biomaterial Properties. Chapman & Hall, London, 341–354
11 Liang K (1990) Contribution a l'étude des mécanismes de fissuration des céramiques de type oxyde. PhD thesis, INSA de Lyon, France
12 Chevalier J, Olagnon C, Fantozzi G. Crack propagation and fatigue in zirconia-based composites. Composites. Part A: applied science and manufacturing 1999; 30: 525–530

4.2 New Generation Ceramics

G. Willmann

Abstract

There are various wear couples that proved to work in total hip replacement: Metal-on-polyethylene, alumina ceramics-on-polyethylene, zirconia ceramics-on-polyethylene and alumina ceramics-on-alumina ceramics. Wear debris is causing particle induced osteolysis and aseptic loosening followed by revision surgery. There is consensus that for long-term application polyethylene should be eliminated in total hip replacement (THR).

Alumina ceramics (BIOLOX®) were introduced nearly 30 years ago as a candidate material for bearing surfaces in THR. The performance and longevity of the joint replacement by virtue of ceramics' inertness and wear resistance are facts. Mg-PSZ zirconia ceramics were introduced about 10 years ago in the USA. It had to be replaced by Y-TZP zirconia ceramics which offer better mechanical strength. All wear couples ceramic-on-PE reduce the PE-wear rates to lower than 0.1 mm per year when comparing to metal-on-PE (more than 0.2 mm per year). For long-term application the wear couple alumina-on-alumina is the most attractive one because of its extremely low wear rate (app. 0.001 mm per year).

The modular femoral-ball concept – i.e. combination of components – is increasing the surgeon's flexibility. Based on this concept, combinations like zirconia-on-alumina are possible. The results of investigations on zirconia-on-alumina are very controversial. Some people report disastrous wear, some do not. From the tribological point of view the wear couple zirconia-on-alumina is close to a high, risky wear mode. We advice not to approve the wear couple zirconia-on-alumina because of zirconia's lack of phase stability.

Today there is even more need to optimize the bearing surfaces in total hip replacement because surgery on young patients has to be performed.

The well known medical-grade ceramics are mono-phase ceramics and brittle. Due to that the risk of fracture cannot be eliminated. The idea is to combine the attractive properties of the various ceramics, i.e. a ceramic composites may solve this problem. A new ceramic biocomposite TTPA (tetragonal toughened platelet reinforced alumina) which is a combination of hard alumina and tough zirconia. It may offer the option to improve the fracture toughness and the mechanical strength (i.e. reliability).

The concept of combining components (modular implant systems) and combining the attractive properties of materials (composite) will surely be the concept in this millennium.

Particle Induced Osteolysis Still is a Problem

The pioneering efforts of John Charnley led to a breakthrough in total hip replacement (THR). About 30 years ago he introduced an artificial joint with a metal femoral head articulating against a cup made of polyethylene (PE-UHMW). Today there are various wear couples that proved to work in clinical application (5,19,24,26,29,34):
- Metal-on-polyethylene (Me/PE),
- alumina ceramics-on-polyethylene (A/PE),
- zirconia ceramics-on-polyethylene (Z/PE) and
- alumina ceramics-on-alumina ceramics (A/A).

Wear debris is causing particle induced osteolysis and aseptic loosening followed by revision surgery. There is consensus that for long-term application polyethylene should be eliminated in THR.

Table 1 Some prerequisites for boinert bioceramics used in THR (5)

Material properties	Offering
Hardness, No plastic deformation, No cold flow	Long-term wear resistance
Finely grained microstructure, No porosity	Excellent surface finish
High strength, Good fatigue properties	Reliability, low risk of fracture
Corrosion resistance	Biocompatibility, bioinertness
Ionic structure, Low contact angle	Wettability, synoviaphilic

Ceramics in THR

Alumina ceramics (Al_2O_3) were introduced nearly 30 years ago as a candidate material for bearing surfaces in THR (Table **1**). It was proven that the performance and longevity of the joint replacement by virtue of ceramic's inertness and wear resistance are facts. Some important prerequisites are:
- excellent corrosion resistance in body environment → biocompatibility
- high hardness → wear resistance
- high Young's modulus, no creep, no cold flow → no deformation
- good wettability, low contact angle → low friction
- good surface finish → low friction
- phase stability → long-term reliability,
- sufficient mechanical strength → reliability, no fatigue

So far more than 2.5 million alumina ceramic heads and more than 100,000 ceramic acetabular components (liners) have been used worldwide. The mostly used ceramic heads and acetabular components (liners) are made of BIOLOX®*forte* manufactured by CeramTec AG, Germany. The 1st generation of ceramic BIOLOX® liners for metal-backed acetabular components was introduced in 1986, the 2nd generation BIOLOX®*forte* liners in 1994 (21). Ceramic liners can be used in combination with more than 50 metal-backed cups.

There are various ceramics that have been developed for bearing surfaces in THR. In Table **2** terms, definitions and important properties are listed.

In the USA the combination ceramic head articulating against polyethylene is a Class II product. Approval is possible based on 510 k. Ceramic wear couples are classified as Class III. 6 Investigational Device Exemptions (IDE) are ongoing (status end of 1999).

Zirconia (ZrO_2) was introduced about 10 years ago in Australia and in the USA (7,11,15). The material used was Mg-PSZ (*p*artially *s*tabilized *z*irconia with *m*agnesium oxide as additive). It had to be replaced by Y-TZP (*t*etragonal *p*olycrystalline *z*irconia stabilized with *y*ttrium oxide). Y-TZP zirconia offers higher mechanical strength than Mg-PSZ (Table **4**).

Zirconia heads are used in combination with PE cups. Zirconia is classified as a Class II product. The first zirconia heads that were approved by the FDA were made of Mg-PSZ. Heads made of Mg-PSZ were offered by the American Company BioPro.

The term "advanced ceramics" describes those products which are ceramics by nature, i.e. inorganic, nonmetallic and sintered polycrystalline solids. These advanced ceramics are based on synthetic raw materials only (no clay). The most important ones are silicon carbide (SiC), silicon nitride (Si_3N_4). All these materials are extremely hard, offer good mechanical strength and corrosion resistance. Material scientists had developed these ceramics for cutting tools, gas turbines and heat engines. Based on screening tests that have been performed for biocompatibility and wear testing (ring-on-disc) it can be concluded that advanced ceramics based on silicon carbide or silicon nitride do not offer sufficient potential for wear couples in THR (20).

The wear couples A/PE and Z/PE reduce the PE-wear rates to lower than 0.1 mm per year when comparing to Me/PE (more than 0.2 mm per year) (5,19,24,34). For long-term application the wear A/A is the most attractive one because it

Table 2 Ceramics in THR: Terms and definitions used

Term	Explanation	Remarks
α-Al_2O_3	corundum, phase of alumina, no phase transformation	stable from low temperatures up to the melting point (3)
A	alumina ceramics	according to ISO 6474, ASTM F 603 and FDA's guidance document
A/A	alumina head articulating against alumina acetabular component (cup)	today's standard
A/PE	alumina head articulating against PE cup	today's standard
Al_2O_3	aluminum oxide = alumina	oxide of aluminum metal
cubic	c-ZrO_2, one of the phases of zirconia	stable at temperatures above 2400 °C (3, 36)
Me	metal	cobalt chrome molybdenum alloy
Me/PE	metal head articulating against PE cup	today's standard
MgO	magnesium oxide = magnesia	oxide of magnesium metal
Mg-PSZ	MgO partially stabilize zirconia	the stabilizer MgO inhibits the phase transformation t → m (3, 36)
Mg-PSZ/PE	Mg-PSZ head articulating against PE cup	
monoclinic	m-ZrO_2, one of the phases of zirconia	stable at low temperatures (3, 36)
PE	polyethylene	today's PE: PE-UHMW
PSZ	partially stabilized zirconia	stabilizer needed, e.g. MgO (3)
SN	abbreviation for various silicon nitrides	advanced ceramics (3)
Si_3N_4	silicon nitride	advanced ceramics (3, 20)
SiC	silicon carbide	advanced ceramics (3, 20)
stabilizer	material needed to stabilize the metastable tetragonal phase of zirconia (t-ZrO_2)	e.g. MgO and Y_2O_3 (3)
tetragonal	t-ZrO_2, one of the phases of zirconia	not stable at room temperature, stable above about 1200 °C (3, 36)
TTPA	app. 75% Al_2O_3, app. 24% ZrO_2 additives Cr_2O_3 and SrO	(4, 14) see papers Kaddick, Pfaff, and Rack in this Proceeding
TTPA/TTPA	TTPA head articulating against TTPA cup	R&D, (14) see papers by Kaddick, Pfaff, and Rack in this Proceeding
TZP	tetragonal polycrystalline zirconia	stabilizer needed, e.g. Y_2O_3
Y_2O_3	yttrium oxide = yttria	oxide of yttrium metal
Y-TZP	Y_2O_3 stabilizes the tetragonal zirconia	the stabilizer yttria (Y_2O_3) inhibits the phase transformation t → m
Y-TZP/PE	Y-TZP head articulating against PE cup	
Z	zirconia ceramics	Y-TZP according to ISO 13356
Z/A	zirconia head articulating against alumina acetabular component	see Table 3 a, b
Z/Z	zirconia head articulating against zirconia acetabular component	see Table 3 a, b
ZrO_2	zirconium oxide = zirconia	oxide of zirconium metal
ZTA	zirconia toughened alumina	advanced ceramics (1, 2, 3, 4)
ZTA/PE	ZTA head articulating against PE cup	R&D (1)
ZTA/ZTA	ZTA head articulating against ZTA cup	R&D (2)

4.2 New Generation Ceramics

Table 3a Wear couples used in THR (5, 19, 21, 23, 29, 33)

Wear couple head/cup	Linear wear rate per year	Comments	Standards available for	Approved by FDA
Me/PE	0.2–0.5 mm	long-term experience, satisfactory clinical results when used for old and not active patients	metal and PE	yes
A/PE	Less than 0.1 mm	Long-term experience, good clinical results	alumina and PE	yes
Mg-PSZ/PE	Less than 0.1 mm	Mid-term experience, good clinical results, not used anymore.	No standard for Mg-PSZ zirconia	yes
Y-TZP/PE	Less than 0.1 mm	Mid-term experience, good clinical results	Y-TZP zirconia	yes
A/A	0.005 mm	Long-term experience, very good clinical results	Alumina and for the wear couple A/A	Class III Product, 6 IDEs ongoing in USA
Z/A	controversial	In vitro test, very few clinical cases	No standard for the wear couple	no

Table 3b Wear couples to be evaluated for THR (1, 2, 14, 20, 24, 30)

Wear couple head/cup	Wear rate	Comments
DLC/PE		not in clinical use
TiN/PE		TiN coating comes off, not used
SiC/x		The biocompatibility of SiC is inferior.
SN/x		The biocompatibility of SN is inferior.
Z/A	Ring-on-disk, roller-on-plate, hip simulator, a few clinical cases	CeramTec does not approve Z/A (9, 17, 33, 35)
Z/Z	In vitro tests only: very controversial reports	CeramTec does not approve Z/Z (33)
ZTA/PE	Hip simulator test only	PE-wear rate: same order as A/PE (1)
ZTA/ZTA	Hip simulator test only	Wear rate lower than A/A (2)
TTPA/TTPA	Hip simulator test only	Wear rate lower than A/A, see Kaddick's paper in this Proceeding

Table 4 Typical values of mechanical properties of bioceramics used in THR or maxifacial surgery

Material	Fracture toughness K_{Ic} in MPa m$^{1/2}$	Mechanical strength in MPa
Bioglass	1	less than 100
Hydroxyapatite (HA)	1	less than 100
Alumina ceramics	4.2	580
Mg-PSZ	8.1	500
Y-TZP zirconia ceramics	up to 10	1 000

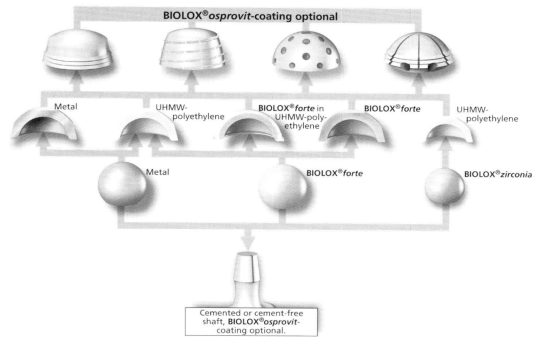

Fig. 1 Modern design concept of THR systems: Combination of components e.g. femoral ball heads made of metal, alumina (BIOLOX®*forte*) or zirconia (BIOLOX®*zirconia*). The heads are fixed on stems by taper fixation. Today's acetabular devices are metal-backed shells with a liner (insert) made of metal, alumina (BIOLOX®*forte*) or polyethylene (PE-UHMW). The stem or the metal shell may be coated with the bioactive hydroxyaptite (BIOLOX®*osprovit*). For comments on approving see Table **4**.

offers the option to overcome the problem of osteolysis due to its extremely low wear rate (Table **3a**).

Today's alumina is hot isostatically pressed (HIP), laser marked and 100% proof-tested (22). Due to that the microstructure is much finer and the mechanical strength is improved. When testing wear couples A/A using this improved material the findings are: less than 0.001 mm per 1 million cycles (23), or less than 0.1 mg per one million cycles. (23, 28, 29).

To summarize (Table **3b**):

1. Mono-phase ceramic heads made of alumina or zirconia articulating against polyethylene reduce wear when compared to metal-on-polyethylene.
2. Alumina-on-alumina offers the lowest wear rates known.
3. There are risks when using the wear couple zirconia-on-alumina.
4. Ceramics based on silicon carbide or silicon nitride do not offer sufficient potential for THR.
5. Mono-phase, high-purity alumina ceramics are the best material known so far, but it is brittle. In THR even fracture rates as low as 0.004% are not accepted by the orthopaedic community.

Approval of Wear Couples

The modular femoral-ball concept increases the surgeon's flexibility. Today a modern THR system consists of a metal stem with metal or ceramic heads that are fixed by taper fixation. The socket is metal-backed with liners made of ceramics, metal or polyethylene (Fig. **1**).

Based on this concept all kinds of combinations are possible. Some combinations are forbidden, e.g. a metal head articulating against a ce-

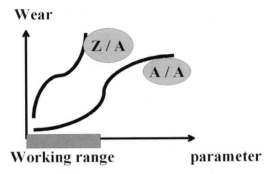

Fig. 2 Wear vs. parameters like sliding velocity, load, lubrication, sphericity or surface finish etc. From the tribological point of view the combination alumina-on-alumina (A/A) is in a low-wear mode when used in THR. The combination zirconia-on-alumina (Z/A) is very close to the high-wear mode.

ramic liner. Ceramics are much harder than metal. If this combination (Me/A) would be used, then a severe metallosis would occur.

The combination zirconia-on-alumina (Z/A) is possible, too. The results of investigations on Z/A are very controversial (9,14,19,31,33). Some people report disastrous wear, some do not. From the tribological point of view Z/A is in or close to a high wear mode (Fig. 2) (35). Due to frictional heating, Hertzian contact stress the phase transformation tetragonal → monoclinic may be triggered. If so there is a volume increase causing stress in the microstructure. Due to that cracks will be initiated, grains will come off and 3rd body wear will occur (9,17,33,35).

Zirconia is a metastable material. Based on material research for heat engines zirconia's hydrothermal instability is well known, i.e. zirconia is not stable when in contact with water (35). Due to the reactions between ZrO_2 or Y_2O_3 and H_2O stress induced cracks can be formed (stress corrosion). Zirconia ceramics are always in humid environment, e.g. humidity in air, water for cleaning (washing) and steam when autoclaving. There were some cases with zirconia heads that had failed in vivo. Therefore the FDA (8) and the British MDA (16) published warnings not to sterilize zirconia in an autoclave. Hydrothermal stability is essential because in hospitals implants will be re-sterilized by steam. So mono-phase alumina offers the best wear and corrosion resistance.

The wear couples approved by FDA are listed in Table **3a**. The FDA is supposed to have the toughest regulations to get approval for implants. Therefore the information if devices were approved by FDA is listed in Table **2**. In the European Community the regulations for approval are different. It is much easier to perform clinical studies and to offer new medical devices to the market. e.g. acetabular components with alumina liners (wear couple A/A). Some people promote the wear couple zirconia-on-alumina (Z/A). CeramTec does not approve the wear couple Z/A and Z/Z because of zirconia's lack of phase stability (33,36) and hydrothermal instability (8,16, 36).

Coatings

There is R & D going on to coat metal components with hard, thin layers, e.g. DLC-coating (*di*amond *l*ike *c*oating) and TiN-coating (*ti*tanium *n*itride) on femoral metal heads. Again the idea is to combine the hardness of TiN and DLC and the good mechanical properties of metal used for heads. DLC-coated heads and TiN-coated heads are combined with polyethylene cups. Some people use the term "ceramic coating". This refers to the basic properties of these coatings, e.g. hard, synoviaphilic, bioinert etc. Up to now there are no satisfactory clinical results proving that these concepts work.

Future Ceramics

There is even more need to optimize the bearing surfaces in THR because surgery on young patients has to be performed. When using ceramics even fracture rates as low as 0.004% (32) are a concern. Long-term reliability became a topic. Mono-phase bioceramics are brittle. Due to that the risk of fracture cannot be eliminated. Modern design (modular design in THR, no monolithic sockets) and advanced ceramic composites may solve this problem.

The ceramic composites are well known for many years. Material scientists are familiar with composites (3,4). In biomaterials this would be a new approach: Ceramic biocomposites like zirconia toughened alumina (1,2,30) and tetragonal toughened platelet reinforced alumina (TTPA) which is based on hard alumina and tough zirconia (Table 2) may offer the option to improve the mechanical strength and the reliability or the in vivo fracture rate. Fracture toughness is a measure for brittleness. If the fracture toughness is low (Table 4) than the material brittle and vice versa. Zirconia has a high fracture toughness, i.e. it is less brittle than alumina.

Toni's team started research evaluating a ceramic heads and cups made of the composite ZTA (zirconia touhgened alumina). Toni's team had tested ZTA heads articulating against PE cups (ZTA/PE) and ZTA heads articulating against ZTA cups (ZTA/ZTA) in a hip simulator varying the zirconia content (1,2). They report that the ZTA-on-PE does not offer a lower wear rate when comparing to alumina-on-PE.

The reason may be that the wear rate of ceramic-on-PE depends on the surface finish of the ceramic head only. Sauer (24) reported the same when comparing the wear rate of Z/PE and A/PE.

CeramTec's solution is to improve the reliability of ceramics in THR by using the advanced biocomposite TTPA. TTPA's trade name will be BIOLOX®delta. The matrix material alumina offers extreme hardness (about 2000 HV, nearly as hard as diamond). When adding zirconia to a matrix this may improve the mechanical strength, the fracture toughness and may reduce the risk of failure. There is a variety of two-phase materials containing intergranular ZrO_2 particles. Small amounts of yttria (Y_2O_3) are usually added to further stabilize the tetragonal phase. BIOLOX®delta (TTPA) is offering a bending strength higher than 1000 MPa. Previous commercial applications of TTPA had been cutting tools.

The advanced ceramic composite BIOLOX®delta contains app. 75% hard alumina and app. 24% tough zirconia. There are additives: Chromium oxide and strontium oxide. BIOLOX®delta is a biocompatible material according to the European standard EN DIN 30993-1 (6). BIOLOX®delta is a bioinert. It is wear resistant. The wear resistance is dominated by the hard alumina grains in the composite. For more details see the papers by Kaddick, Pfaff, and Rack in this Proceedings.

The wear rate vs. zirconia content was tested using the ring-on-disk test and hip simulator. For the composition mentioned above BIOLOX®-delta-on-BIOLOX®delta (TTPA/TTPA) (14). the wear rate was lower than the one for standard alumina-on-alumina (23).

So far all results prove that the concept of using BIOLOX®delta (TTPA) may be superior to the well known mono-phase ceramics alumina or Y-TZP zirconia. For more test results see the papers by Kaddick, Pfaff, and Rack in this Proceedings.

Conclusion

Long-term clinical experience and future options are summarized in Table 5:

Table 5 What's out? What's in? What may be next?

Biomaterials/Application for THR	Out	In	Next
Monolithic alumina cups	*		
Ceramic stems	*		
Alumina ceramics in contact with bone	*		
THR: Modular design		*	
Wear couple: alumina heads and polyethylene cup (A/PE)		*	
Wear couple: Y-TZP heads and polyethylene cup (Y-TZP/PE)		*	
Femoral Mg-PSZ heads (Mg-PSZ/PE)	*		
Alumina liners for acetabular components		*	
Y-TZP liners for acetabular components	*		
Wear couple: alumina head and alumina liner (A/A)		*	
Wear couple: zirconia head and alumina liner (Z/A)	*		
Composite: Bioinert hard coatings on metal, e. g. DLC or TiN			?
Advanced ceramics: silicon nitride, silicon carbide	*		
Biocomposite TTPA: TTPA head and polyethylene (TTPA/PE)			*
Biocomposite TTPA: TTPA head and TTPA liner (TTPA/TTPA)			*

1. Ceramic heads made of mono-phase alumina or zirconia ceramics that articulate against polyethylene (A/PE, Z/PE respectively) reduce wear by a factor of two when compared to metal-on-polyethylene (Me/PE).
2. Mg-PSZ zirconia has been replaced by Y-TZP zirconia due to its better mechanical strength.
3. Y-TZP zirconia does not offer sufficient hydrothermal stability. It shall not be sterilized with steam.
4. Alumina-on-alumina (A/A) offers the lowest wear rates known (0.001 mm per year).
5. There are risks when using the wear couple zirconia-on-alumina (Z/A) because of Y-TZP's insufficient phase stability. CeramTec does not approve the wear couple zirconia-on-alumina (Z/A).
6. Mono-phase, high-purity alumina ceramics are the best material known so far, but it is brittle. In THR even fracture rates as low as 0.004% are not accepted by the orthopaedic community. A new approach may be a ceramic biocomposite.

A new approach to optimize ceramics for bearing surfaces is a composite combining alumina's attractive properties, its hardness and zirconia's, its toughness. The new ceramic biocomposite TTPA (tetragonal toughened platelet reinforced alumina, trade name BIOLOX®*delta*) may offer option to improve the reliability of ceramic heads and acetabular components. It is expected the TTPA/PE and TTPA/TTPA offer wear rates better than A/PE and A/A, respectively. Kaddick, Pfaff, and Rack will report on the results of various investigations on the advanced biocomposite TTPA in this Proceedings.

The options we have in R&D are the
- **combining** components in THR (the modular design concept)
- **combining** good material properties, i.e. **composites.**

The advanced biocomposite TTPA (BIOLOX®*delta*) may offer the option to reduce the risk of failure. More R&D on this advanced biocomposite will be performed in this millennium.

References

1 Affato S, Testoni M, Cacciari GL, Toni A (1999) Mixed oxides prosthetic ceramic ball heads. Part 1. Effect of the ZrO_2 fraction on the wear of ceramic on polyethylene joints. Biomaterials 20: 971–975
2 Affato S, Testoni M, Cacciari GL, Toni A (1999) Mixed oxides prosthetic ceramic ball heads. Part 2. Effect of the ZrO_2 fraction on the wear of ceramic on ceramic joints. Biomaterials 20: 971–975
3 Brook RJ (1991) Concicise Encyclopedia of Advanced Ceramic Materials. Pergamon Press, Oxford
4 Burger W. Umwandlungs- und plateletverstärkte Aluminiumoxidmatrixwerkstoffe. (1997) Part 1: Keram. Z. 49: 1067–1070 (1998) Part 2: Keram. Z. 50: 18–22
5 Clarke I, Willmann G (1994) Structural Ceramics in Orthopedics. In: Cameron HU (ed): Bone Implant Interface. Mosby, St. Louis, 203–252
6 DIN EN 30,993: Biological evaluation of medical devices. European Standard, 1994
7 Fishman G, Clare A, Hench L (1995): Bioceramics: Materials and Application. Ceramic Transactions Vol. 48, The American Ceramic Society, Westerville
8 Food and Drug Administration (1997) Steam Re-Sterilization Causes Deterioration of Zirconia Ceramic Heads of Total Hip Prostheses. http://www.fda.gov/cdrh/steamst.html Food and Drug Administration, Washington DC, USA
9 Früh HJ, Willmann G, Pfaff HG (1997) Wear Characteristic of Ceramic-on-ceramic for Hip Endoprostheses. Biomaterials 18: 873–876
10 Garino JP (1998) Design Considerations and Preliminary Results with the Wright Medical "Transcend" Acetabular Cup System. In: Puhl W (ed): Bioceramics in Orthopaedics – New Applications. Enke Verlag, Stuttgart, 39–43
11 Huckstep RL, Lutton PP (1991) New Concepts in Stabilization and Replacement of Bones and Joints. Materials Forum 15: 252–260
12 ISO-Norm 13,356 (1997) Implants for surgery – Ceramic materials based on yttria-stabilized tetragonal zirconia (Y-TZP). International Standard Organization
13 ISO 6474 (1994) Implants for surgery – Ceramic materials based on high purity alumina. International Standard Organization

14 Kaddick C, Pfaff HG (1999) Wear Study on the Alumina-zirconia System. In: Sedel L, Willmann G: Reliability and Long-term Results of Ceramics in Orthopaedics. Georg Thieme Verlag, Stuttgart, 93–98

15 Litton PP, Huckster RL, Howell CR (1993) Modular Ceramic and titanium Locking Devices in Orthopedic Surgery. J AST Cream Soc. 29: 91–102

16 Medical Device Agency Adverse Incident Center (1996) Zirconia ceramic heads for modular total hip femoral component: Advice to users on resterilization. Medical Device Agency Adverse Incident Center, Safety Notice MDA SN 97,617

17 Morlock MM, Nassutt R, Honl M, Janßen R, Willmann G (1999) The wear couple zirconia/alumina in a hip joint: a case study. In: Sedel L, Willmann G (1999) Reliability and Long-term Results of Ceramics in Orthopaedics. Georg Thieme Verlag, Stuttgart, 99–104

19 Morscher EW (1995) Endoprosthetics. Springer Verlag, Berlin

20 Orth J, Macedo S, Wilke A, Griss P (1992) Osseointegration of Hydroxyapatite-Coated and Uncoated Bulk Alumina implants in the Femur of Göttingen Minipigs-Mechanical Testing of Bonding Strength. In: Ravaglioli A, Krajewski A (1992) Bioceramics and the Human Body. Elsevier Appl Sci, London, 302–307

21 Puhl W (1998) Biocermics in Orthopaedics – New Applications. Enke Verlag, Stuttgart

22 Richter HG, Willmann G (1999) Reliability of Ceramic Components for Total Hip Prostheses. Brit Ceram Trans 98: 29–34

23 Saikko V, Pfaff HG (1998) Low wear and friction in alumina/alumina total hip joints: A hip simulator study. Acta Orthop Scand 69: 443–448

24 Sauer WL, Anthony ME (1998) Predicting the Clinical Wear Performance of Orthopaedic Bearing Surfaces. In: Jacobs J, Craig T L (1998) Alternative Bearing Surfaces in Total Joint Replacement. STP 1346, American Society for Testing Materials, West Conshohocke, PA, USA 1–29

25 Sedel L, Cabanela ME (1998) Hip Surgery – Materials and Developments. Martin Dunitz, London

26 Sedel L, Willmann G (1999) Reliability and Long-term Results of Ceramics in Orthopaedics. Georg Thieme Verlag, Stuttgart

27 Siverhus SW (1998) Design Considerations and Preliminary Results with the Wright Medical Osteonics. Acetabular Cup System. In: Puhl W (1998) Biocermics in Orthopaedics – New Applications. Enke Verlag, Stuttgart, 2–6

28 Taylor SK, Serekian P, Manley M (1998) Wear Performance of a Contemporary Alumina – alumina Bearing Couple Under Hip Joint Simulation. 44th Ann. Meeting, ORS, March 15–19, 1998 New Orleans, Louisiana, 51–9

29 Taylor S (1999) In-vitro Wear Performance of a Contemporary Alumina: Alumina Bearing Couple under Anatomically – relevant Hip Joint Simulation. In: Sedel L, Willmann G (1999) Reliability and Long-term Results of Ceramics in Orthopaedics. Georg Thieme Verlag, Stuttgart

30 Toni A (1999) New Wear Couples for THR – Simulator Testing. In: Sedel L, Willmann G (1999) Reliability and Long-term Results of Ceramics in Orthopaedics. Georg Thieme Verlag, Stuttgart, 84–86

31 Villermaux F, Blaise L, Drouin J M, Cales B (1998) Ceramic – ceramic Bearing Systems for THP with Zirconia Heads. Bioceramics 11: 73–76

32 Willmann G, von Chamier W (1998) The Improvements of the Materials Properties of BIOLOX Offer Benefits for THR. In: Puhl W (1998) Bioceramics in Orthopaedics – New Applications. Enke Verlag, Stuttgart, 19–24

33 Willmann G, Frueh HJ, Pfaff HG (1996) Wear Characteristics of Sliding Pairs of Zirconia (Y-TZP) for Hip Endoprostheses. Biomaterials 17: 2157–2162

34 Willmann G (1998) Ceramics for Total Hip Replacement – What a Surgeon Should Know. Orthopaedics 21: 173–177

35 Woydt M, Kadoori J, Habig K H, Hausner H (1991) Unlubricated Sliding Behavior of Various Zirconia-based Ceramics. J European Ceramic Soc 7: 135–145

36 Yashimura M (1988) Phase Stability of Zirconia. Bull Amer Ceram Soc 67: 1950–55

4.3 A New Material Concept for Bioceramics in Orthopedics

H.-G. Pfaff, R. Rack

Introduction

Hip arthroplasty has been developed to a very common procedure. Surgical techniques, medical treatment and implant technology contributed to increased survivorship of implants. The expectation of the patient has changed from being free of pain to regaining unlimited mobility for a long term. The progress in the implant technology is associated with the development and introduction of new biomaterials.

In modern implant technology the combination of components out of different materials in modular components is very common. All materials used have a special performance profile. The analysis of these profiles suggests that there is no optimal material (Table **1**).

Regarding this list, the question may be raised, is there an application for another ceramic material? The development of orthopedics in the 90's focused on the problem of wear debris induced osteolysis, and improved wear couples were introduced into orthopedics.

For high demand applications, metal on metal as well as ceramic on ceramic bearings, a new market segment emerged [1]. The use of metal on metal bearings is still associated with the question of allergic and carcinogenic reactions, which are not definitely answered [2]. Based on the very promising clinical application of ceramic bearings the demand in ceramic bearings increases rapidly. Zirconia materials now being used clinically for ten years, reveal problems due to the poor hydrothermal stability [3,4]. Recently offered zirconia on alumina bearings can not be considered as safe bearings, as with increasing phase transformation, the wear couple fails; alumina however has a limited strength, therefore the application remains limited to designs with sufficient wall thickness. Thus, there is a strong need in a new bearing material that paces a further development in arthroplasty such as small

Table 1 Materials in orthopedics

Material	Application	Advantage	Limitation
CoCr Alloys	Stems, cups, wearing surfaces	High strength, good wear material against UHMWPE metal on metal bearing	Biological reactions on wear debris not clear, allergic reactions
Titanium alloys	Implant components contacting bone	Good bioacompatibility high strength	No bearing surface material,
Alumina	Wear components	Excellent wear resistance against itself and UHMWPE	Strength limitations, failure mode
Zirconia	Wear components against UHMWPE	Excellent strength	Chemical resistance, not autoclavable, failure mode
Hydroxylapatite	Coating material	Bioactive	Poor strength
UHMW PE	Wear components	Wear material against metal and ceramic	Strength, biological reaction on wear debris, creep resistance
PMMA	Bone cement	High strength cement, biological inert	Fatigue resistance

diameter bearings or ceramic liners with elevated rim.

Many ceramic materials are being considered for use in wear applications. Siliconnitride materials for instance are materials of the first choice, regarding high strength and toughness. But these materials fail as wear resistant bearing materials in the configuration of total hip replacements [5].

As alumina offers advantages like chemical resistance, excellent bioinertness even in the form of wear debris [6], and wear resistance, the development of a new material has to include alumina as a matrix material.

Further the inertness of the material against all sterilization procedures is required. The strength properties including Weibull's modulus are to exceed the existing materials.

Concepts of Improving Ceramics

In material science materials are described by different parameters. The term toughness is used in a different meaning regarding ceramics and metals. A tough metal means that the metal can be plastically deformed prior to the failure. Plastic deformation is the shifting of lattice layers that dissipates energy. Tough ceramics mean that the material has a high resistance against crack propagation under stress (Figs. **1, 2**).

In fracture mechanics of ceramics, the relationship between toughness and strength is given as

$$\sigma = \frac{K_{1c}}{\sqrt{a}} \cdot y$$

with σ = strength
K_{1c} = fracture toughness
a = flaw size
y = material constant

To improve the strength of a ceramic material, toughness and flaw size are both parameters to be considered.

As flaw size and grain size of the microstructure are associated with each other, a reduction of the grain size contributes as well to a gain in strength. The development of Biolox alumina ceramics highlights this relationship [7]. But with the introduction of the HIP process, that revealed a improved microstructure, the potential for further significant improvements of alumina ceramics has diminished.

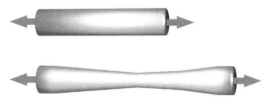

Fig. 1 Toughness of metal materials is the resistance against plastic deformation.

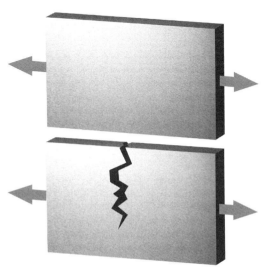

Fig. 2 Toughness of ceramics is the resistance against crack growth.

In the late 70's the principle of transformation toughening as a mean to improve the strength of alumina matrix materials was developed [8]. Small particles, e.g. zirconia, were finely dispersed in an alumina matrix. As zirconia is not a thermodynamically stable material, a phase transformation at 1170 °C occurs from the monoclinic to the tetragonal phase. The phase transformation is associated with decrease in volume. Therefor in the cooling down phase, the volume increases. Small particles in the matrix can remain in the high temperature phase if the particles are well encapsulated in the alumina matrix. The transformation occurs only if a crack touches the particle. This process dissipates energy that would otherwise be used for crack growth and contributes therefore to a increased toughness (Fig. **3**).

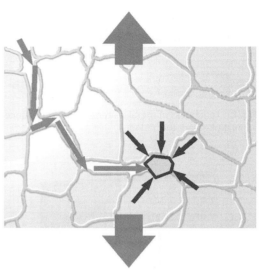

Fig. 3 The principle of transformation toughening by zirconia particles, which are dispersed in the alumina matrix.

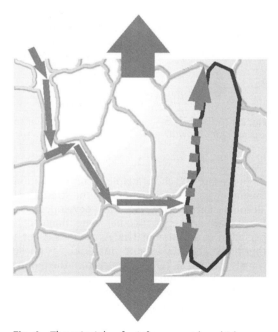

Fig. 4 The principle of reinforcement by whiskers or plateletlike crystals in a alumina matrix.

These ZTA (zirconia toughened aluminas) never found their way into medical application. Any gains in toughness had to be paid off with a lower Weibull's modulus. That makes the material very questionable for long term high demand applications. Thus the reliability of the material was not considered to be appropriate and research into ZTA ceramics was abandoned.

Another approach to improve strength is the principle of reinforcement by introducing anisotropic crystals like whiskers. Other than in metals or in plastic composits, where ceramic fibers are embedded in a matrix with a low elastic modulus, in a ceramic matrix the elastic moduli of fibers and matrix are relatively similar. Therefor the mechanism of toughening is different (Fig. **4**).

The crack energy is dissipated by the deviation of the crack around the fiber crystal, which is associated with an increase in strength and toughness. This material concept however did not produce alumina based materials for commercial applications, as the technological problems could not be overcome successfully.

The challenge of the development of a new ceramic material was to overcome the above mentioned problems and as the described concepts did not reveal a major improvement, to explore concepts that leave the existing findings behind.

Transformation Toughened and Platelet Reinforced Alumina: An Alumina Matrix Composite

The complex requirements as described above cannot be met with single phase materials, therefore more complex material systems had to be explored. Based on the long term experience with ZTA systems [9] and the development of coated Y-TZP ceramics [10], in the ZTA system two major advantages could be achieved.

By the introduction of Yttria-coated nano-sized zirconia particles, the existing problems of ZTA ceramics could be overcome. The coating technology enables to shift the strength maximum towards higher zirconia contents, as the transformation kinetic is now more controlled, and not stochastic as with uncoated zirconia particles. At the same time the toughness can be raised significantly. Higher amounts of zirconia however reduce the hardness of the material which is not desirable for any medical wear resistant material. Cromiumoxid and alumina form solid solutions and the addition of cromiumoxid increases the hardness of alumina. With the dotation of cromiumoxid in the alumina ma-

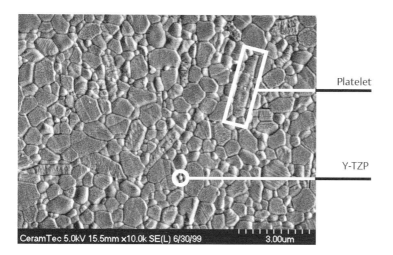

Fig. 5 Microstructure of the alumina matrix composit Biolox Delta.

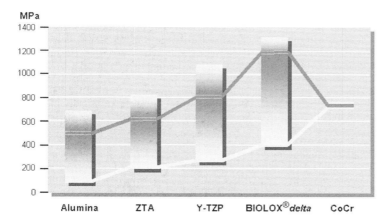

Fig. 6 Whereas metals are characterized by minimum values, ceramists use mean values. The lower line is a calculated allowable stress for ceramics, to make both material groups comparable.

trix the drop in hardness can be compensated. However the gain of hardness is associated with a drop in toughness, therefore another composit had to be added [11].

The addition of SrO to alumina forms platelet like crystals. A controlled introduction can achieve the in-situ generation of stontiumaluminat platelet crystals in the matrix during the sintering process giving these particles excellent fixation in the alumina matrix.

The advantage of this in situ generation of platelets is the more homogenous distribution and superior size distribution as an addition of platelet crystals into the powder.

The influence of the platelets on strength and toughness is enormous. A high strength material with high hardness and high toughness can be achieved.

Being aware of the complexity of the parameters of this pentary system the possibility of the development of a taylored medical grade material was given, meeting or exceeding the mentioned requirements (Fig. **5**).

The Advantage of the New Material

It has always been a vision of the material scientists to combine the properties of metals and ceramics. Despite of the fact that the failure mode of ceramics, which is fracture, cannot be changed with the development of this Alumina Matrix

Composite (AMC) material the properties of ceramics could be shifted significantly into the direction of metal (Fig. **6**).

Due to the improved strength and strength distribution the allowable stress level in a component can be raised by the order of one magnitude. This offers new degrees of freedom in the design. The existing limits of diameters and wall thickness need to be redefined. Applications like knee components are now technically feasible.

The new possibilities suggest the excellent clinical performance of alumina ceramics in hip arthroplasty can now be transferred to fields of applications where components out of existing material do not meet the expectations of the surgeon.

References

1 Black J.: Prospects for Alternate Bearing Surfaces in Total Replacement Arthroplasty of the Hip, Performance of the Wear Couple BIOLOX forte in Hip Arthroplasty, Enke, Stuttgart 1997
2 Amstutz Harlan C. et al: Metal on Metal Total Hip Replacement Workshop Consensus Document, Clinical Orthopaedics and Related Research Number 329 S, Lippincott-Raven Publishers, 1996
3 Le Mouel S.: Premiers résultats alarmants du couple zyrcon/polyéthylène dans les prothèses totales de hanche. Abstract: Revue de Chirurgie Orthopédique et réparatrice de l'appareil moteur, 72ᵉ Réunion annuelle de la Société Française de Chirurgie Orthopédique et Traumatologique, 44, 1997
4 Chevalier J., J. M. Drouin, B. Cales: Low temperature aging behaviour of zirconia hip joint heads, in: Sedel L., Ch. Rey (ed.): Bioceramics 10. Pergamon, Elsevier Sci. Ltd., Oxford, 1997, p.135–138
5 Kaddick Ch.: Versuchsbericht 1999
6 Henßge, E. J., I. Bos, G. Willmann: Al_2O_2 against Al_2O_2 combination in hip endoprotheses. Histologic investigations with semiqantitative grading of revision and autopsy cases and abrasion measures. J. Mt. Sci. Mat. in Medicine 5 (1994) 657–661
7 Willmann G., W. von Chamier: The Improvements of the Material Properties of BIOLOX Offer Benefits for THR, Bioceramics in Orthopaedics – New Applications, Enke, Stuttgart, 1998
8 Claussen N.: Fracture Toughness of Al_2O_3 with an Ustabilized ZrO_2 Dispersed Phase, Journal of The American Ceramic Society, Vol. 59, No. 1–2
9 Dworak U., H. Olapinski, G. Thamerus: Festigkeitssteigerung von mehrphasigen keramischen Werkstoffen am Beispiel der Systeme ZrO_2-ZrO_2/Al_2O_3-ZrO_2/Al_2O_3-TiC. Ber. DKG 55 (1978) 98–101
10 W. Burger: Zirkonoxid in der Medizintechnik. In: Technische Keramische Werkstoffe, Hrsg.: J. Kriegesmann in Zusammenarbeit mit der DKG, 1996, Kapitel 8.7.2.0, 15–25
11 W. Burger: Umwandlungs- und Plateletverstärkte Aluminiumoxidmatrixwerkstoffe (Teil 1 und 2), in: Keramische Zeitschrift 49 (12) 1997

4.4 A New Ceramic Material for Orthopaedics

R. Rack, H.-G. Pfaff

Introduction

For more than 25 years the name Biolox®*forte* stood for excellent quality and performance "made in Germany" in orthopaedic implants. This high performance material has been created to conform the need of physicians for inert and wear resistant components for hip joint replacement. Today, Biolox®*forte* is in many countries the standard material used. Performance of these wear couples is based upon the following criteria:
- Excellent biocompatibility
- No ion release/no allergic responses
- Good mechanical performance
- Chemical/hydrothermal stability
- Superior tribology/wear results

Excellent clinical results have been the reported [1], and they have effectively made Biolox®*forte* the golden choice for a very large number of indications. Today, more than 2.5 million components have been implanted, mainly in 28 mm and larger wear couples.

In recent years, the use of Zirconia has been promoted as the natural step in ceramics evolution. The higher strength characteristics are supposed to enable finer designs, while keeping the excellent results of bio-inertia and wear resistance. Unfortunately, the complex nature of Zirconia has to this day caused much uncertainty on the material's ability to perform well, especially under hydrothermally challenging conditions during sterilisation or even in vivo [2].

Recent literature reports first trails with mixed Alumina – Zirconia ceramics showing promising in vitro results [3]. These "new" ZTA materials have been used in mechanical applications for more than 20 years; their use as biomaterials is relatively new. Now a new development has managed to combine the positive effects of Alumina and Zirconia ceramics, while abstaining from negative influences by the latter partner. This new material – TTPA (transformation toughened and platelet reinforced Alumina) promises excellent mechanical performance from the Zirconia parent, while avoiding the problems of hydrothermally induced degradation through the use of an Alumina matrix material.

Why are these new and promising materials not already in use today? The demands from regulatory bodies and the user – be it surgeon or patient – are extremely high. The material is to be used in a long-time application in one of the most difficult environments, the human body. Therefore it is necessary to absolutely assure the safety and performance of the product. Thus many different series of tests and essays have to be undertaken to characterise the material and minimalise all risks, before the material can be considered "safe" for implantation trails.

Biocompatibility

The testing of all materials to be used in implantation has been regulated in Europe by the international standard ISO 10993 (see Table **1**). Countries outside the continent require specific testing procedures, usually governed by a local body, like the US FDA, or the Japanese MHW, although they share the same approach [4]. The number and nature of the tests are related to the biomaterial's use. As an implant device in permanent (> 30 days) contact with bone and tissue, like the wear couple for hip joint replacement, AMC requires the following biological evaluations:

A cytotoxicity test according to ISO 10993-5 has been performed on crushed material as well as an wear debris by a GLP laboratory and no cell-toxically harmful substances have been found.

Taking the use of AMC as a permanent implantable device, the chemical composition of a

Table 1 Tests for Biological Evaluation of Materials (acc. to ISO 10993-1) and testing results of Biolox®forte (Alumina) and Biolox®delta (AMC)

Biological Effect	Biolox®forte	Biolox®delta
Cytotoxicity	+	+
Sensitisation	+	+
Genotoxicity	+	+
Implantation	+	+
Chronic Toxicity	+	+
Carcinogenicity	+	+

AMC eluate served as a base for an assessment on the following biological effects: sensitisation, genotoxicity and carcinogenicity, irritation of tissue in direct contact, systemic and subchronical toxicity. No release of trace ingredients in toxicologically relevant concentrations could be found.

With the success of these tests, an series of implantation trails in rats and rabbits have been performed. The subcutaneous, intra-muscular and intra-osseous implantation of AMC particles produced only a slight local irritant effect in the implantation sites after implantation periods of 4 weeks and 6 months.

On the basis of these results, it can be concluded that the abraded material is tolerated after long-lasting contact with tissues [5]. So far, no implantation tests have been done on human patients.

Mechanical Characterisation

AMC is an Alumina matrix material, tailored to high performance in the orthopaedics domain. To start the mechanical qualification program a series of tests have been performed according to a international standards. These showed the results depicted in Table **2**, below.

Some values are specific data used by ceramists to characterise ceramic materials, and can be translated into more commonly used terms, like

Table 2 Average values of Biolox®delta and other bioceramics

Material Properties	Units & Standards	Biolox®forte (Alumina)	Biolox®zirconia (Y-TZP)	ZTA ceramic material [3]	Biolox®delta (AMC)
Density	g/cm³ DIN EN 623-3	3980	6040	5020	4365
Colour	– –	ivory	off white	off white	mauve
Young's Modulus	GPa DIN EN 843-2	380	210	285	350
Poisson's Ratio	– DIN EN 843-2	0.23	0.3	0.25	0.22
Flexural Strength	MPa DIN EN 843-1	580	1050	912	1150
Weibull's Modulus	– DIN V ENV 843-5	5	10	7	13
Compressive Strength	MPa ASTM C695	5000	2200	–	4700
Fracture Toughness	MPam$^{1/2}$ (notched beam)	4.3	10.5	6.9	8.5
Hardness	HV0,5 DIN V ENV 843-4	2300HV0,5	1250HV0,5	1500HV1	1975HV1
Thermal Stress Factor	K (calculated value)	203	304	–	317
Water Absorption	% ASTM C373	0	0	–	0
Wetting Angle	° –	water: 45 Ringer's: 5	Ringer's: 10	–	Ringer's: 2.5

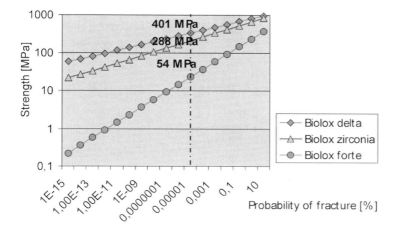

Fig. 1 Strength of biomaterials calculated from Weibull's distribution.

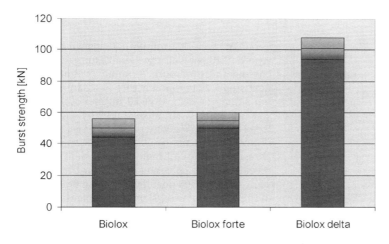

Fig. 2 Development of burst strength (and standard deviation) of ballheads 28 – 12/14 L.

reliability or (inverted) probability of failure by the use of the Weibull's distribution:

$$F(\sigma_{4PB}) = 1 - e^{-\left(\frac{\sigma_{4PB}}{\sigma_0}\right)^m}$$

The high value of flexural strength σ_{4PB} of 1150 MPa, coupled with a high "reliability coefficient", the Weibull's modulus m give an increased security against fracture of the ballhead. The calculated stress value at a 0.0004% risk of fracture is 401 MPa (in comparison, Biolox®forte shows 54 MPa strength, while Biolox®zirconia reaches 288 MPa, see Fig. 1). Therefore the theoretical safety factor against fracture of the AMC component has been raised by 7 to 8. But there are many other factors, ranging from the surgeon's performance to the patient's sportive habits, that greatly influence the result of a prosthesis and also the wear couple. So it is necessary to take a closer look at the components:

The results can be transported onto the Biolox®delta ballhead, as depicted in Fig. 2. High burst strength values of 100 kN or more are also common when testing e.g. Zirconia ballheads. Unfortunately, these high strength materials have a severe weakness limiting their clinical use – they are complex multi-phasic materials that are not inherently stable at ambient temperature. Generally, this effect is used to make the component more resistant to fracture (a so-called transformation toughening effect), but it can be triggered involuntarily under hydrothermal conditions, like the autoclave [6] or even in vivo [7]. AMC has been tested under the severe conditions of multiple cycles in the Autoclave and shows no

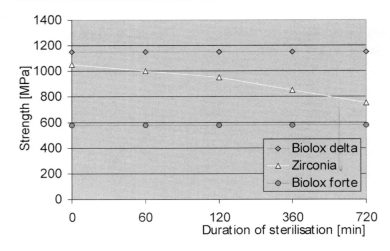

Fig. 3 Hydrothermal ageing (by Autoclave) of biomaterials.

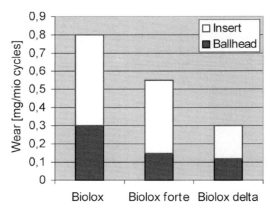

Fig. 4 Performance of wear couples from the Biolox product range.

strength degradation (see Fig. 3). Further samples have been artificially aged before undergoing a hip simulator study for 10 million cycles, without notable difference in result from its virgin brethren. It can therefore be concluded that Biolox®-delta is an adept material for high performance applications.

Tribological Data

When it comes to researching materials for a wear couple, one starts out with many different possibilities and has them undergo different tests, always discarding samples that give non-acceptable results. The testing runs performed at CeramTec were started with a ring-on-disc test, where AMC showed excellent results (even surpassing those of pure Alumina ceramics). The next step was to manufacture first samples for a hip simulator test. After 10 million cycles there was minimal wear measurable by gravimetry (see Fig. 4), while geometry and surface topology of the components could not detect any trace of abrasion. The use of high powered SEM imaging revealed slight polishing effects on the surface, such as those well documented from Biolox®forte in the hip simulator [8] or after explantation [9]. The retrieved wear particles were geometrically analysed to evaluate their harmful potential, but found to correspond to the profile know from Biolox®forte wear debris – a reliable and clinically proven tribo-material [10].

Even when using hydrothermally pre-aged samples no relevant difference to the aforementioned excellent results were detected.

A luxation wear test (sliding the ballhead over the insert's rim and back) was used to demonstrate the performance of the new material in this, one of the worst known wear situations. The ballhead could be slid over the rim for 300 times before any difference was noted by the fine-tuned data acquisition device; more than 400 luxation cycles had to be done before a slight roughened spot could be detected on the insert. After 1000 cycles the test was stopped without any visible damage to the ballhead, and only a slight marring of the insert's rim.

With these tests, Biolox®*delta* can be proven to be an excellent sliding couple.

Comparison with Other Bioceramics

In many aspects AMC is characterised by its ceramic nature. When comparing Biolox®*delta* to other bioceramics, one quickly notes that the material not only combines the excellent results of biomaterials like Biolox®*forte* (Alumina) and Biolox®*zirconia*, but also surpasses them in many aspects. These synergetic effects have been known for some time, and thus ZTA materials have been used in mechanical or engineering applications for more than 20 years. In the field of bioceramics, these materials are relatively new, but first tests have shown that their use in orthopaedics could be realisable [3]. But when these Zirconia-rich materials are compared directly to Biolox®-*delta*, they lag behind in critical areas (see Table 2).

Conclusion on Biolox®*delta*

In order to introduce the new ceramic TTPA (transformation toughened and platelet reinforced Alumina) to the orthopaedic arena, the material has to be very well documented and tested:

Biocompatibility testing according to ISO 10993 was successful: No harmful effects were found.

Mechanical characterisation showed excellent results, surpassing those of known bioceramics like Alumina and Zirconia, and even new developments like ZTA ceramics for orthopaedics.

The tribological situation of Biolox®*delta* (AMC) was examined, especially under the challenging conditions of hydrothermal ageing. The results documented the aptitude of this material in wear applications, from ring on disc tests to hip joint simulation.

Thus AMC has proven itself to be a ceramic material of superb abilities for orthopaedic use.

Possibilities with Biolox®*delta* are many-fold, the door for new applications has been pushed wide open!

References

1. Puhl W. (ed) (1997) Performance of the Wear Couple BIOLOX forte in Hip Athroplasty. Enke
2. Chevalier J., Drouin J. K., Cales B., (1997) Low Temperature Aging Behaviour of Zirconia Hip Joint Heads. Bioceramics 10: 135–138
3. Toni A., Affotato S. (1999) New Wear Couple for THR – Simulator Testing in: Sedel L., Willmann G. (eds) Reliability and Long-term Results of Ceramics in Orthopaedics. Thieme: 82–85
4. Black J. (1999) Biological Performance of Materials – Fundamentals of Biocompatibility. Dekker
5. Dannhorn D. (1999) Evaluation of Local Tolerance of Abraded Material in Implantation Tests over 6 Months in Rabbits. Ochsenhausen
6. Food and Drug Administration (1997) Steam Re-Sterilization Causes Deterioration of Zirconia Ceramic Heads of Total Hip Protheses. http://www.fda.gov/cdrh/steamst.html
7. Pfaff H.-G., Willmann G. (1998) Stability of Y-TZP Zirconia, in: W. Puhl (ed), Bioceramics in Orthopaedics – New applications. Enke: 29–31
8. Taylor S. K. (1999) In-vitro Wear Performance of a Contemporary Alumina: Alumina Bearing Couple Under Anatomically-Relevant Hip Joint Simulation, in: Sedel L, Willmann G. (eds) Reliability and Long-term Results of Ceramics in Orthopaedics, Thieme: 85–90
9. Prudhommeaux F, Nevelos J, Doyle C., Meunier A., Sedel L. (1998) Analysis of Wear Behaviour of Alumina – Alumina Hip Protheses after 10 Years of Implantation. Bioceramics 11: 621–624
10. Böhler M., Mochida Y., Bauer T. W., Salzer M (1999) Analysis of Wear Debris Particles from Alumina on Alumina Ceramic THA, in: Sedel L, Willmann G. (eds) Reliability and Long-term Results of Ceramics in Orthopaedics, Thieme: 57–59

4.5 Wear Study in the Alumina-Zirconia System

C. Kaddick, H.-G. Pfaff

Introduction

The past decade of ceramic developments has been characterized by investigations about biocompatibility, strength and wear resistance of alumina as well as zirconia components. Corresponding to the initial phase of metals used for surgery, the questions have been focused on the developments of pure materials known from other technical applications.

The world of ceramics becomes much more complex by introducing mixtures of different elements like alumina and zirconia. Besides the fact that the strength of the new material has to be as good or even better than the established ones, the wear resistance of those composites can not be predicted by theoretical calculations.

To minimize time and costs, a simple screening test has to be used separating the huge number of imaginable material combinations into approved candidates and abortive developments. This test series has to be followed by an additional mechanical test as close as possible to the in-vivo conditions. It is generally agreed that using a ring-on-disc test according to ISO 6474 followed by hip simulator tests is a sufficient method to follow the above mentioned procedure.

Part 1 of this investigation has already been published [6]. As a results, a mixture of 75% alumina and 24% zirconia proved to be one of the most promising composites. It therefore has been decided to manufacture implants to be tested in a hip simulator to enable comparison to the materials in clinical use right now.

Materials and Methods

A total of three ceramic inserts and balls made of a composite of alumina and zirconia (Table 1) with a nominal diameter of 28 mm and +0 mm

Table 1 Material properties

Al_2O_3 content	75%
$ZrO_2 + Y_2O_3$-content	24%
Cr_2O_3	0.3%
SrO	0.8%
bending strength	1150 MPa
hardness	1975 HV1
density	4.365 g/cm^3

neck extension have been tested. The sphericity deviation has been equal or less than 7 µm.

The inserts were fixed using a titanium metal shell as already in clinical use.

The simulator used performs movement of all in-vivo axis according to the normative references. The orientation of the implant is "anatomic correct" using an inclination of 10° between the axis of the insert and the axis of the ball. The load direction is kept constant versus the ball. The tests have been performed according to ISO TR 9325 and ISO TR 9326.

The resulting hip joint force is applied by a computerized servo hydraulic system. The cup is fixed on a swivel arm responsible for the flexion/extension as well as the abduction/adduction movement. Rotational movements are applied versus the fixation of the ball (Fig. **2**).

All tests are performed under bovine serum according to Table **2**. No attempt has been made to externally heat the serum to 37 °C. Routine measurements of the temperature indicated a range of 34 °C to 36 °C after temperature settlement.

Wear has been calculated by weight loss using a high precision balance which provides a 0.01 mg standard deviation about the average weight of the ceramic components.

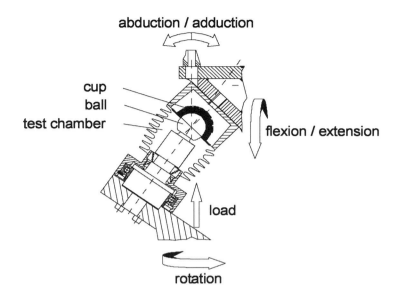

Fig. 1 Position of the specimens and kinematics of the simulator.

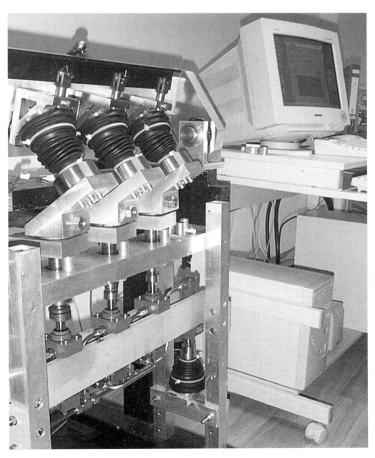

Fig. 2 Three-station hip simulator used.

Table 2 Test parameters

axial load	double-peak according to BERGMANN
load maximum	2.5 kN
Frequency	1.0 Hz
angle applied load/cup	45°
angle cup/insert	10°
flexion-extension	± 25°
abduction-adduction	± 10°
Rotation	± 10°
test fluid	bovine serum
Cycles	3 Mio.
inspection cycles	500,000

Table 3 Lubricant (400 ml)

serum	100 ml
Amphotericin	4 ml
EDTA	2.338 g
auqa dest.	rest to 400 ml

The test has been stopped at intervals of 500,000 cycles to replace the serum and to gain the actual weight of the specimens.

The couplings have been changed periodically between the three stations.

The protein content of the undiluted serum has been 60.77 g/l resulting in a lubricant protein content of 15.19 g/l.

After test finish, SEM of the bearing surfaces has been performed.

Results

As indicated in Fig. 3, a run-in period up to 0.5 Mio cycles has been observed. The total amount of wear after 10 Mio cycles has been 0.7 mg (StdDev 0.03 mg) for the balls and 1.0 mg (StdDev 0.10 mg) for the cups.

Assuming 1 Mio cycles per year, a linear wear rate of 0.06 mg/year (StdDev < 0.001 mg/year) for the balls and 0.09 mg/year (StdDev 0.006 mg/year) for the cups can be calculated.

SEM of the bearing surfaces

Non-worn surfaces are predominantly featureless. As indicated in Fig. 4, occasional pores and

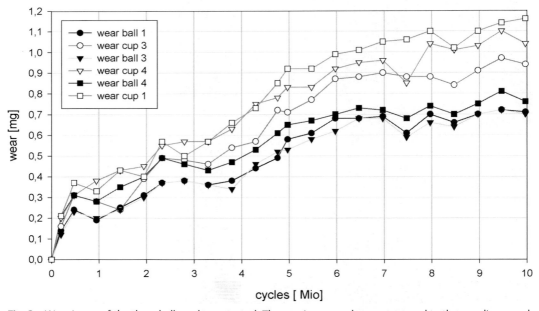

Fig. 3 Wear in mg of the three balls and cups tested. The specimen numbers correspond to the couplings used.

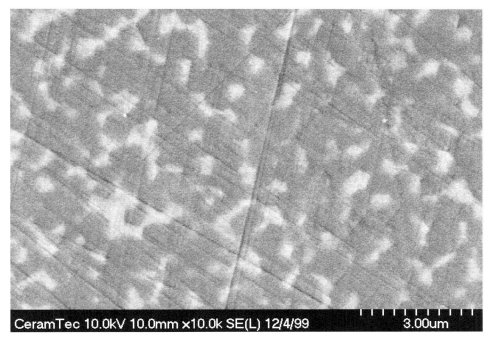

Fig. 4 SEM of ball #1 after 10 Mio cycles.

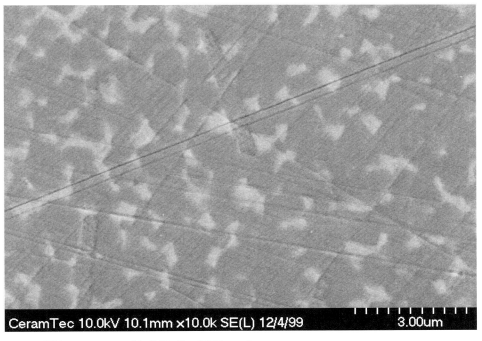

Fig. 5 SEM contact area of ball #1 after 10 Mio cycles.

Table 4 Calculated wear rates for 1 Mio cycles

Specimen	wear rate [mg/year]
Insert 1	0.10
Insert 3	0.09
Insert 4	0.09
Ball 1	0.06
Ball 3	0.06
Ball 4	0.06

polishing marks can be observed. Focussing the SEM onto the rarely seen worn areas, smooth abrasion (Fig. 5) as well as scratching can be observed. No signs of grain pull-out could be detected. Scratches following the kinematics of the simulator as well as irregular scratching are found. In comparison to alumina bearing surfaces, which show very few wear marks, the surfaces of the new material show even less and smaller wear marks. This in addition supports the hypothesis that the wear resistance of the new material is superior to the established alumina.

Discussion

The lack of clinical data about in-vivo wear of ceramic bearings hinders the validation of hip simulator results. Due to the fact that wear rates of polyethylene vs. ceramic have been reproduced by the simulator used in this study, the kinematics as well as the loading can be regarded to be approved. Previous tests using pure alumina ceramic components (Biolox-forte) are within the range of published data gained by other investigators [2,7,9], some of them using different setups.

No attempt has been made to investigate the influence of the test fluid onto the wear rates. Although the composition of the serum used herein is widely accepted to represent the synovial fluid [3], an impact of the composition itself can not be excluded an needs further investigation.

To predict the biological impact of the of the wear reduction between Biolox-forte and Biolox-delta, the particle size generated has to be taken into consideration [1,10]. Up to now, particle analysis according to ISO/WD 17853 [5] could not be performed sufficiently. This may be related to the small particle size expected from SEM observations.

Comparing the wear rates ratio between the insert and the balls results in about 3:2. It is assumed that this factor is related to the different loading paths of the components: Whereas the applied force acts at the same point of the ball, the insert is moving relatively to the load. Upcoming ISO regulations [3,4] will standardize the simulators in use worldwide to enhance reproducibility as well as to enable direct comparison between the different test laboratories.

References

1. Campbell P et al.: Isolation of predominantly sub-micron-sized UHMWPE wear particles from periprothesic tissues. J. Biomed. Mat. Res. 29 (1995) 127–131
2. Fisher et al.: Wear and debris generation in artificial hip joints. in: Reliability and long-term results of ceramics in orthopaedics. Sedel L, Willmann G, ed. Thieme, Stuttgart, 1999
3. ISO/DIS 14242-1: 1999-06: Implants for surgery – wear of total hip prostheses – Part 1: Loading and displacement parameters for wear-testing machines and corresponding environmental conditions for tests.
4. ISO/DIS 14242-2: 1998-11: Implants for surgery – wear of total hip prostheses Part 2: Methods of measurement
5. ISO/WD 17853: Method for the isolation, characterization and quantification of polymer and metal wear debris.
6. Kaddick, C. Pfaff H. G.: Wear study in the alumina-zirconia system. in: Reliability and long-term results of ceramics in orthopaedics. Sedel L, Willmann G, ed. Thieme, Stuttgart, 1999
7. Oonishi, H. et al.: Investigation of the wear behavior of ceramic on ceramic combinations in total hip prostheses. Bioceramics Vol 9 (1993) 503–506
8. Taylor, S. K.: In-vitro wear performance of a contemporary alumina: Alumina bearing couple under anatomically-relevant hip joint simulation. in: Reliability and long-term results of ceramics in orthopaedics. Sedel L, Willmann G, ed. Thieme, Stuttgart, 1999
9. Walter, A.: On the material and the tribology of alumina-alumina couplings for hip joint prostheses. Clin Ortho Rel Res 282 (1992) 31–46
10. Wirth, M. A. et al.: Isolisation and characterization of polyethylene wear debris associated with osteolysis following total shoulder arthroplasty. J. Bone Joint. Surg. 81-A (1999) 29–37

5 CeramTec Award 2000

5.1 CeramTec Award 2000

At the occasion of the International Symposiums in Stuttgart, Germany CeramTec has awarded a prize for outstanding studies with regard to the problems of wear in total joint replacment. This prize shall be awarded to young surgeons, engineers, or scientists who published or submitted as a publication or thesis these research results in the field of wear couple in orthopaedics.

For the CeramTec Award 2000 lots of good papers had been submitted. There were papers on clinical investigations and papers on technical topics, too. The papers were evaluated by
- Prof. Springorum (Bad Mergentheim, Germany)
- Prof. Stock (Braunschweig, Germany)
- Prof. Zichner (Frankfurt, Germany)
- PD Dr. Willmann (Plochingen, Germany)

The committee decided that J. E. Nevelos' paper was the best one, J. Huber's and S. Affato's papers were second, they had the same score.

J. E. Nevelos (U.K.)
Wear of HIPed and Non-HIPed Alumina-Alumina Hip Joints Under Standard and Severe Simulator Testing Conditions (Abstract see next page).

J. Huber (Germany)
Optimierung von Gleitpaarungen für künstliche Gelenke.

S. Affatato (Italy)
Mixed-oxides prosthetic ceramic ball heads.
Part 1: Effect of the ZrO_2 fraction on the wear of ceramic on polyethylene joints
Part 2: effect of the ZrO_2 fraction on the wear of ceramic on ceramic joints.

5.2 Wear of HIPed and Non-HIPed Alumina-Alumina Hip Joints Under Standard and Severe Simulator Testing Conditions

J. E. Nevelos, E. Ingham, C. Doyle, A. B. Nevelos, J. Fisher

Abstract

Wear and wear debris of artificial hip joints remain major concerns in total hip arthroplasty (THA). The long term effects of UHMWPE wear debris are well documented and these have led to interest in alternate bearing materials for THA. Alumina ceramic-ceramic hip joints have been successfully used for nearly thirty years with low wear and little incidence of osteolysis. The most common wear pattern observed on retrieved components is an elliptical wear 'stripe' on the heads and a corresponding worn area on the cup with an approximated wear rate of 1–5 mm^3 per annum. More severe wear has also occasionally occurred, usually in association with an abnormal clinical history. Modern alumina-alumina THAs use an improved HIPed alumina ceramic bearing material which may be more resistant to severe wear. Previous *in vitro* simulator studies have not replicated *in vivo* wear rates or mechanisms. The aim of this study was to compare previous generation non-HIPed alumina and modern HIPed (hot isostatically pressed) alumina in a physiological hip joint simulator under 'normal' and 'harsh' testing conditions.

HIPed alumina was found to have a lower wear rate than non-HIPed alumina, although the difference was not statistically significant. Testing in Gelofusine® and water lubricants had no effect on the wear rates of either material. Elevated swing phase load testing also had no significant effect on the wear rates of either material. Testing in the absence of any lubricant produced very severe wear of the non-HIPed material in one specimen only.

Key words: Ceramic – Total Hip Arthroplasty – Wear – Hip Simulator

5.3 CeramTec Award 1996 – 1999

The winner of the previous CeramTec Awards had been:

1999 **Prudhommeaux F. (Paris, France)**
with the paper "Analysis of Alumina – alumina Hip Prostheses Wear Behavior after 10 Years of Implantation" submitted to Clin. Orthop. Rel. Res.

1998 **Lu, Z., H. McKellop (Los Angeles, USA)**
with the paper "Frictional heating of bearing materials tested in a hip joint simulator"
Proc. Instn. mech. Engrs 211 Part H (1997) 101 – 108

1997 **Th. Lindenfeld (Frankfurt, Germany)**
"In vivo Verschleiß der Gleitpaarungen Keramik – Polyethylen gegen Metall – Polyethylen. [In vivo wear of the wear couples ceramics-on-polyethylene and metal-on-polyethylene]"
Orthopäde 26 (1997) 129 – 134

1996 **E. Fritsch (Homburg/Saar, Germany)**
"Biocompatibility of Alumina – Ceramic in Total Hip Repalcement. Macroscopic – and Microscopic Findings on capsular Tissues after Long-term Implantation"
In: W. Puhl (1996) Die Keramikpaarung BIOLOX in der Hüftendoprothetik [The ceramic Wear Couple BIOLOX in Total Hip Replacement] Enke Verlag, Stuttgart, 12 – 17

6 Suggested Reading

6.1 Suggested Reading

G. Willmann

Bioceramics in Orthopaedics

Since the 1970's when first it was realized that the properties of alumina ceramics could be exploited to provide better implants for orthopedic applications, the field has expanded enormously. Initial applications depended on the fact that alumina ceramics were bioinert and provided wear characteristics suitable for bearing surfaces.

Resultant orthopedic use has enjoyed nearly 30 years' clinical success, e.g. BIOLOX®forte alumina femoral heads, sockets, and acetabular liners for total hip replacement. About 10 years ago zirconia was approved for use as femoral ball heads articulating against polyethylene cups. The bioactive hydroxyaptite offers attractive tissue reactions. It is well established as coating on metal implants to enhance osseointegration. Hydroxyapatite (HA) is used for bone grafting, too.

The bioceramics mentioned are commercially used in Northern America, Japan, Australia, and Europe. There are lots of publications, Reviews, and books about application of bioceramics. I had compiled some important references in:

Willmann G (1998) A Bibliography of Published Literature on Bioceramics for THR. In: Puhl W (1998) Bioceramics in Orthopaedics – New Applications. Enke Verlag, Stuttgart, 132–136

Willmann G (1999) A Bibliography of Published Literature on Bioceramics for THR: 1st Update. in: Sedel L, Willmann G (1999) Reliability and Long-term Results of Ceramics in Orthopaedics. Georg Thieme Verlag, Stuttgart, 114–117

Suggested Reading

Biomaterials is an expanding field. There are lots of papers, too much to compile all. Therefore I list a selection of some of the latest publications which may be worth reading.

There are more and more reports on zirconia's hydrothermal instability and lack of phase stability. The second part of this review is a list of papers reporting on problems with Y-TZP zirconia ceramics. Based on this information we are discussing to stop manufacturing and offering Y-TZP zirconia for medical applications.

Some Reviews

Various Authors (1999) Chapter 2: Ceramics for Joints. in: Ogushi H, Hastings GW, Yosjikawa T (1999) Bioceramics 12. World Scientific, Singapore, New Jersey, London 61–102

Bensmann G (1999) An Attempt to Assess Material Suitability Taking the Example of Hip Endoprostheses. Materialwiss u Werkstofftechnik 30: 733–745

Black J (1988) Does Corrosion Matter? J Bone Joint Surgery 70 B: 517–520

Black J, Hastings G (1998) Handbook of Biomaterial Properties. Chapman & Hall, London

Black J (1999) Biological Performance of Materials – Fundamentals of Biocompatibilty. Marcel Dekker, Inc. New York, Basel, Hong Kong

Costa L, Brach del Prever EM (2000) UHMWPE Polyethylene for Arthroplasty: Characterization, Sterilization and Degradation. Edizioni Minerva Medica, Torino

Havelin LI (1999) The Norwegian Arthroplasty Register. In: Jacob R, Fulford P, Horan F (1999) European Instructional Course Lectures Vol 4. The British Editorial Society of Bone and Joint Surgery, London, 88–95

Helsen JA, Breme HJ (1998) Metals as Biomaterials. John Wiley & Sons, Chichester, New York, Weinheim

Heros R, Willmann G (1998) Ceramics in Total Hip Arthroplasty: History, Mechanical Properties, Clinical results and Current Manufacturing State of the Art. Seminars of Arthroplasty 9: 114–122

Jacobs JJ, Craig ThL (1998) Alternative Bearing Surfaces in Total Joint Replacement. STP 1346, ASTM, West Conshohocke, PA, USA

Jacob R, Fulford P, Horan F (1999) European Instructional Course Lectures Vol 4. The British Editorial Society of Bone and Joint Surgery, London

Jenisson HP (1999) Biomaterials. Materialwiss u Werkstofftechnik 30, special issue No 12

Oonishi H, Amino H, Ueno M, Yunoki H (1999) Concepts and Designs with Ceramics for Total Hip and Knee Replacement. in: Sedel L, Willmann G (ed.) Reliability and Long-term Results of Ceramics in Orthopaedics, Georg Thieme Verlag Stuttgart, 7–28

Ogushi H, W Hastings G, Yosjikawa T (1999) Bioceramics 12. World Scientific, Singapore, New Jersey, London

Piconi C, Maccauro G (1999) Zirconia as a Biomaterial. Biomaterials 20: 1–25

Puhl W (1996) Die Keramikpaarung BIOLOX in der Hüftendoprothetik. Proc 1st Symposium in Stuttgart, March 23, 1996, Enke Verlag, Stuttgart

Puhl W (1997) Performance of the Wear Couple BIOLOX forte in Hip Arthroplasty. Proc 2nd Symposium in Stuttgart, March 8, 1997, Enke Verlag, Stuttgart

Puhl W (1998) Bioceramics in Orthopaedics – New Applications. Proc 3rd Symposium in Stuttgart, Feb 14, 1998, Enke Verlag, Stuttgart

Sedel L, Cabanela M E (1998) Hip Surgery – Materials and Developments. Martin Dunitz, London

Sedel L, Willmann G (1999) Reliability and Long-term Results of Ceramics in Orthopaedics. Georg Thieme Verlag, Stuttgart

Schmalzried TP, McKellop H (1999) Polyethylene primar: Manufacturers work to improve polyethylene for hip prostheses. Orthopedics today Int. ed. 2 Nov/Dec, 14–17

Springorum HW, Trutnau A, Braun K (1998) Fachlexikon Orthopädie – Hüfte. ecomed Verlagsges mbH Landsberg/Lech

Williams FD (1992) Medical and Dental Materials. VCH, Weinheim

Willert HG, Buchhorn GH (1999) The Biology of the Loosening of Hip Implants. In: Jacob R, Fulford P, Horan F (1999) European Instructional Course Lectures Vol 4. The British Editorial Society of Bone and Joint Surgery, London, 58–82

Willmann G, Ceramic Acetabular Cups for Total Hip Replacement. Part 1–8. Biomed Technik 41 (1996) 98–105; 41 (1996) 284–290; 42 (1997) 256–263; 43 (1998) 184–186; 43 (1998) 342–349; 44 (1999) 345–351; 44 (1999) 345–351; 45 (2000) in print

Willmann G (1999) Ceramics for Joint Replacement: What is the Options for the next Millennium? Interceram 48 (1999) 389–397

Willmann G (1999) Coating of Implants with Hydroxyapatite – an Option for the Establishment of Positive Material Connections between Bone and Metal. Adv Eng Mat 1: 95–105

Willmann G (2000) Bioceramics in Orthopaedics: What did we learn in 25 years? [Biokeramik in der Orthopädie – Was haben wir aus 25 Jahren gelernt?] Med Orth Tech 122: 10–16

Wintermantel E, Ha SW (1998) Biokompatible Werkstoffe und Bauweisen Implantate für Medizin und Umwelt 2. Auflage. Springer Verlag, Berlin, Heidelberg, New York

Wise DL, Trantolo DJ, Altobelli DE, Yazemski MJ, Gresser JD, Schwartz ER(1995) Encyclopedic Handbook of Biomaterials and Bioengineering. Marcel Dekker, New York, Basel, Hong Kong

Zirconia

Allain J, Le Mouel S, Goutallier D, Voisin MC (1999) Poor eight-year survival of cemented zirconia – polyethylene total hip replacement. J Bone Joint Surgery 81 B: 835–842

Amin KA, Nag D (1995) Tribological Characteristics of Zirconia – Yttria Ceramics. Bull American Ceramic Soc 74: 80–84

Food and Drug Administration (FDA) (1997) Steam Re-Sterilization Causes Deterioration of zirconia Ceramic Heads of Total Hip Prostheses. http://www.fda.gov/cdrh/steamst.html (FDA) Food and Drug Administration

Früh HJ, Willmann G, Pfaff HG (1997) Wear Characteristic of Ceramic-on-ceramic for Hip Endoprostheses. Biomaterials 18: 873–876

Huber M, Lintner F (1999) Bacterial adhesion to femoral ballhead surfaces of artificial hipjoints in vitro. Eur J Orthop Traumatol 9: 245–250

Kaddick C, Pfaff HG (1999) Wear study on the alumina – zirconia system. pages in: Sedel, L. G. Willmann (1999) Reliability and Long-term Results of Ceramics in Orthopaedics, Georg Thieme Verlag, Stuttgart, 96–101

Lu Z, McKellop H (1997) Frictional heating of bearing materials tested in a hip joint simulator. Proc Instn. mech. Engrs 211 Part H: 101–108

6.1 Suggested Reading

Medical Device Agency Adverse Incident Center (MDA) (1996) Zirconia ceramic heads for modular total hip femoral component: Advice to users on resterilization. Medical Device Agency Adverse Incident Center, Safety Notice MDA SN 97,617

Morlock MM, Nassutt R, Honl M, Janssen R, Willmann G (1999) The Wear Couple Zirconia/Alumina in THR: A Case Study. In: Sedel L, G Willmann (1999) Reliability and Long-term Results of Ceramics in Orthopaedics. Georg Thieme Verlag, Stuttgart, 102–107

Murakami T, Ohtsuki N (1992) Friction and Wear Characteristic of Sliding Pairs of Bioceramics and Polyethylene: Influence of Aging on Tribological Behavior on Tetragonal Zirconia Polycrystals. Bioceramics 5: 365–372

Murakami T, Doi S (1999) Influence of Operating Conditions and Material Combinations on Friction and Wear Properties of Ceramic-on-ceramic Sliding Pairs. Bioceramics 12: 71–74

Pfaff HG, Willmann G (1998) Stability of Y-TZP Zirconia. In: Puhl W (1998) Bioceramics in Orthopaedics – New Applications, Enke Verlag, Stuttgart 29–31

Richter HG, Burger W, Osthues F (1994) Zirconia for Medical Implants – The Role of Strength Properties. Bioceramics 7: 401–406

Willmann G, Früh HJ, Pfaff HG (1996) Wear Characteristics of Sliding Pairs of Zirconia (Y-TZP) for Hip Endoprostheses. Biomaterials 17: 2157–2162

Willmann G (1997) BIOLOX®*forte* heads an Cup Inserts for THR – What a Surgeon Should Know. In: Puhl W (1997) Performance of the Wear Couple BIOLOX®*forte* in Hip Arthroplasty. Enke Verlag, Stuttgart, 105–116

Woydt M, Kadoori J, Habig KH, Hausner H (1991) Unlubricated Sliding Behavior of Various Zirconia – based ceramics. J European Ceramic Soc 7: 135–145

Yashimura M (1988) Phase Stability of Zirconia. Bull Amer Ceram Soc 67: 1950–55

Zolotar MS, Zavaglia CAC (1996) Fracture toughness and microstructure degradation of Y-TZP in aqueous physiological environment. Journal of Materials Science – Materials in Medicine 7: 367–369

7 Workshop on the 5th Symposium

7.1 Workshop on the 5th Symposium

G. Willmann

At the occasion of the 5th International CeramTec Symposium **Bioceramics in Hip Joint Replacement** reliability of ceramic femoral heads and ceramic acetabular components (liners, inserts) used in modular system for total hip replacement was one of the topics. Reliability is closely correlated to handling ceramic components and to the range of motion (ROM). On the workshop on Feb. 18, 2000 these topics were discussed and posters were presented.

The posters presented at the workshop and some comments will be made available in summer 2000.[1]

- Ballhead & Taper: Specification (R. Rack)
- Ballhead: Protection Cap (R. Rack)
- Can Ceramic Heads be Used on Damaged Tapers? (H.-G. Pfaff)
- CeramTec's Recommendations for Revision when Using BIOLOX®*forte* Femoral Heads (G. Willmann)
- CeramTec's OP-Chart
- CeraLock®: Insertion Instrument (U. Bunz)
- Know Your Possibilities: The CeraLock® Modular Insert System (U. Bunz)
- How to Deal with Misaligned Liners (H.-G. Pfaff)
- How to Seat a Ceralock® Insert by Hand (U. Bunz)
- Wear Couples in Hip Arthroplasty (H.-G. Pfaff)
- Problems with Zirconia Ceramics for Articulating Surfaces (G. Willmann)
- Range of Motion vs. Impingement (R. Bader/G. Willmann)
- Range of Motion vs. Position and Design (R. Bader/G. Willmann)
- Range of Motion vs. Wear (R. Bader/G. Willmann)
- Range of Motion vs. Dislocation (R. Bader/G. Willmann)

---

[1] Contact CeramTec AG, Medical Products Division, Fabrikstr. 23 – 29, 73207 Plochingen, Germany